Simple Skin
Beauty

Simple Skin
Beauty

Every Woman's Guide to a Lifetime

of Healthy, Gorgeous Skin

Ellen Marmur, MD

with Gina Way

ATRIA BOOKS

New York London Toronto Sydney

Note to Readers

This publication contains the opinions and ideas of its author. It is sold with the understanding that the author and publisher are not engaged in rendering health services in the book. The reader should consult his or her own medical and health providers as appropriate before adopting any of the suggestions in this book or drawing inferences from it.

The author and publisher specifically disclaim all responsibility for any liability, loss or risk, personal or otherwise, which is incurred as a consequence, directly or indirectly, of the use and application of any of the contents of this book.

 ATRIA BOOKS

A Division of Simon & Schuster, Inc.
1230 Avenue of the Americas
New York, NY 10020

Copyright © 2009 by Dr. Ellen Marmur

All rights reserved, including the right to reproduce this book or portions thereof in any form whatsoever. For information address Atria Books Subsidiary Rights Department, 1230 Avenue of the Americas, New York, NY 10020

First Atria Books hardcover edition September 2009

ATRIA BOOKS and colophon are trademarks of Simon & Schuster, Inc.

ssb and colophon are registered trademarks of Ellen Marmur, MD

For information about special discounts for bulk purchases, please contact Simon & Schuster Special Sales at 1-866-506-1949 or business@simonandschuster.com.

The Simon & Schuster Speakers Bureau can bring authors to your live event. For more information or to book an event, contact the Simon & Schuster Speakers Bureau at 1-866-248-3049 or visit our website at www.simonspeakers.com.

Designed by Jaime Putorti
Illustrations by Amy Saidens

Manufactured in the United States of America

10   9   8   7   6   5   4   3   2   1

Library of Congress Cataloging-in-Publication Data

Marmur, Ellen.
  Simple skin beauty : every woman's guide to a lifetime of healthy, gorgeous skin / By Ellen Marmur; with Gina Way.
    p. cm.
  1. Skin—Care and hygiene. 2. Beauty, Personal. 3. Women—Health and hygiene.
  I. Way, Gina. II. Title.
    RL87.M347 2009
    646.7'26—dc22

ISBN 978-1-4165-8696-8
ISBN 978-1-4165-8714-9 (ebook)

*To my patients who inspired me to write this book because of
their passion for knowledge.*

*To my adorable four children and my amazing husband,
my life.*

*To my beloved parents—
the apple doesn't fall far from the tree.*

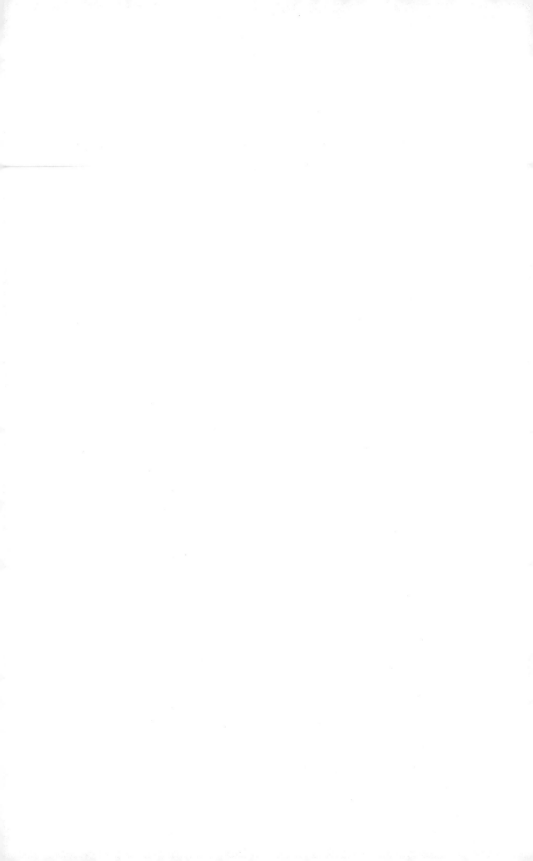

Contents

<u>part three</u>

Regaining Your Youthful Skin

Introduction

Imagine that your best friend is a dermatologist, someone you trust who can help you navigate through the maze of skin care products and dermatologic procedures; someone who will lead you away from purchasing overpriced products unlikely to make a meaningful change in your appearance and let you know which are really worth the money. What would you ask her? What do you really need to use on your skin every day? How can you fight off the lines and brown spots that come with aging, but still look natural—a rejuvenated (but not artificial) version of yourself? Are prescription-strength topical products more effective than the over-the-counter ones, and what will really work for you? Can all these scary-sounding procedures turn back time on your face and body? Are they even safe? Where should you begin?

As the Chief of Dermatologic and Cosmetic Surgery at the Mount Sinai Medical Center in New York City, I specialize in skin cancer surgery, cosmetic surgery and women's health dermatology. My practice is 100 percent academic, so although I see patients full time, I also lecture, teach, and do research. After working on melanoma research at New York University Medical Center and graduating with the highest honor of Alpha Omega Alpha medical society from the Albert Einstein College of Medicine, I completed training in internal medicine at Mount Sinai Hospital and dermatology residency at New York Weill

Cornell Medical Center and Memorial Sloan-Kettering Cancer Center in New York City. Finally, I completed a fellowship in procedural dermatology to specialize in skin cancer surgery, laser surgery, and cosmetic surgery under the mentorship of Dr. David Goldberg. In the past five years, I have published numerous original contributions in peer-reviewed academic journals and delivered lectures on skin cancer and cosmetic surgery at academic meetings nationally and internationally. Presently I train eleven (incredibly bright) residents in dermatologic surgery, direct a procedural dermatology fellowship, co-direct an Advanced Dermatologic Surgery International Fellowship at Mount Sinai, and co-direct an annual dermatology symposium at Mount Sinai. Thus I'm on the cutting edge of the field and can offer my patients (and you) creative, simple skin care solutions.

Every day in my practice, bewildered patients come in and ask the same questions again and again: "Do I really need to wear sunscreen every day, even if it's cloudy?" "How do I use this serum?" "Will this cream make my wrinkles go away?" I realize that there's a message about how to use all these products that's not being heard or understood. What it takes to maintain healthy skin is actually pretty simple: a few basic essentials (a gentle cleanser, a moisturizer, and—if nothing else—sunblock are key) and the know-how to adjust your regimen appropriately to treat issues such as breakouts, dry skin, or both. The store shelves filled with cosmetic products are enticing—and confusing and expensive. The bottom line is most of those creams and potions are unnecessary. Even so, $45 billion is spent in the United States annually on cosmetics and toiletries, and the global market for beauty and personal care products is estimated to be about $360 billion. Given the thousands of choices available (and all that money being spent), some straightforward guidance will help you choose what will work best for your skin—and avoid wasting money on what won't.

I know that "simple" skin care actually seems very complex. And the facts change every day as new ingredients, products, and procedures become available to the public. Few of us have the time, energy, or desire to research hundreds of product ingredients, and only a doctor or a beauty editor can keep track of the latest skin breakthroughs when there seems to be a new laser coming out every month.

I want you to be better educated about your own skin than the person behind the beauty counter or the marketing departments of huge cosmetic companies that are trying to sell a miracle cream. I'll admit that I love to use luxurious beauty products too and fully appreciate the power of feeling good about how you look. As a doctor and mother of four children, I understand that we don't have the time, budget, or patience for beauty nonsense. Because I'm also a skin cancer survivor, I know firsthand how important it is to give your skin the care and attention it deserves. It can actually save your life.

I'll break the facts down in a clear, efficient way and give you straight advice. The same kind I give my patients. Whether you're twenty or eighty, you should start with a simple skin care plan. I think only three or four products are essential, and believe me, the less you use, the better your skin will behave. I'll explain why and teach you how to become your own dermatologist in a sense. Once you learn to read your ever-changing complexion (and it does fluctuate every day), you can troubleshoot skin problems that arise, such as acne flare-ups, rosacea, or dry patches.

I'll help you make sense of the amazing, albeit overwhelming, medical possibilities available to you. Which cosmetic laser can zap brown spots, and which one eliminates redness? Which injectable fillers work best on different parts of your face, neck, hands, and beyond? Is Botox safe? If you start these procedures, will you ever be able to stop?

Diving into the world of cosmetic procedures and cosmeceuticals can feel a little like Alice falling down the rabbit hole into a confusing, surreal new world, where everything from mushrooms and powerful berries to laser beams can be used on your skin. But it doesn't have to be so complicated and perplexing if you understand the basics about how your skin functions. For example, since not much can get past its elaborately durable surface, how can products that promise "cell turnover" and "collagen building" really work? In this book I examine the safety and efficacy of skin care products and cosmeceuticals and investigate whether or not they actually penetrate the skin. Can potentially toxic chemicals such as parabens actually get to the dermis and enter the bloodstream? By the same token, can active ingredients, such as green tea or the new CoffeeBerry, break through the surface of the skin and accomplish their claimed antiaging benefits? These are significant questions and ones that I'm still investigating myself. They are key queries that will be posed throughout this book. *How* products work is something we should ask ourselves when considering the safety and success of anything we put on our skin.

Consider this book an owner's manual for your skin, and refer to it whenever you need dermatologic guidance. Learn what products you should use regularly and what you can add to your regimen to remedy specific skin concerns. Find out how a dermatologist can treat many of these complaints (such as acne and rosacea), and use the multiple medical procedures available to tackle the inevitable issues of aging skin.

By the way, you will see that I mention many products by name in this book. It's important to say I am not a paid spokesperson for any product and have no financial interest in them. Also, please be sure to let a dermatologist see your skin every year, especially when you are using advice from the problems and solutions section of the book, just to be sure your diagnosis and the doctor's diagnosis agree.

In the following pages I'll answer a host of medical and cosmetic questions asked by real women (and men) of all ages across the country. No doubt quite a few are your queries too. How do I know if this freckle is skin cancer? How often should I get a facial? Are extractions safe? What kind of sunblock should I use on my dark skin? What will happen if I don't use sunscreen? What, besides plastic surgery, can help my sagging neck? My answers may surprise you. I'll debunk falsehoods about skin that we take at face value. For instance: you can get skin cancer only from the sun. Not true.

What I love most about being a doctor is coming up with resourceful solutions, solving problems in a simple but inspired way. This is what medical knowledge can offer. After studying philosophy at Vassar College, I learned emergency medical training in order to lead canoe trips in the wilderness. One day a fourteen-year-old girl fractured her ankle. I broke a canoe paddle in half and used some duct tape to splint her leg, then evacuated her twenty-eight miles to the nearest ranger station to be helicoptered out. That moment of breaking the paddle and taping her ankle was one of the most powerful hands-on applications of knowledge that I'd ever experienced, and it instantly changed my life. It made me want to be a doctor.

Currently, I am the principal investigator on more than ten studies. My academic research spans from an FDA safety study using a cosmetic filler in patients with skin of color to Phase II and III clinical trials on new immunomodulatory therapies for skin cancer, varicella zoster virus, and psoriasis. I am also often asked to interpret cosmeceutical claims to the press in magazines and television. As a doctor, what I do is practical and science-based, and I want to pass along that straightforward know-how. As a woman keenly aware of my aging skin and my history of skin cancer, I want us to find that Holy Grail, that perfect antiaging serum! But it must be based on truth and real science. So if your best friend were a dermatologist, what would you ask her? I'm here to tell you what you want—and need—to know.

Ellen S. Marmur

part one

>>> THE BASICS

Know Your Skin and How to Care for It

1

How Your Skin Works

You've already flipped to the chapter on Botox, haven't you? Did you check out the section on what to do for sagging skin and then come back here to the beginning? I don't blame you. Lasers, needles, and antiaging antidotes definitely sound more exciting than an anatomy lesson at first. But knowing how your skin works is not just fascinating (and I don't say that just because I'm a doctor), it is integral to understanding how to care for your complexion, to make it healthier, happier, and ultimately beautiful. So avoid the temptation to skip this section completely and move on to all the juicy stuff about fillers and high-tech products. Since knowledge is power, this is truly the empowerment chapter. With this foundation, everything that follows—about protecting your skin, about cancers and other specific skin conditions, even about cosmetic procedures and products—will make sense. You'll know why many of us have oily T-zones, why most substances can't penetrate into the skin, and why a tan is a bad thing.

After buying a new appliance, a television, or a computer, who actually reads the instruction manual? Usually we just wing it and then dig up the information later when something breaks down or a problem arises. These next few pages are the crucial part of the manual that shows you where everything is and how all the moving parts work. Knowing how your skin operates will help you understand why it reacts the way it does to things such as the sun, what we eat, how well we sleep, and what we put on it.

Try to forget all the boring diagrams and complicated scientific descriptions from your old high school textbooks. The daily workings of the skin are more akin to a thrilling adventure story, filled with bad guys (the sun, infections, and more), special agents (the cells), and high-tech communication systems. Though the skin may appear to be just a pretty, or sometimes problematic, wrapper for the body, there's a lot going on just beneath the surface.

With its intricate framework of layers, vascular system, different kinds of cells and glands, the skin is a miniuniverse. It's amazing the way the body communicates through the microstructures that are set up. When I read my kids *Horton Hears a Who!*, the Dr. Seuss tale of an elephant that discovers a fully functioning yet microscopic planet on a speck of dust, I'm reminded of the amazing, dynamic composition of the skin. If there were a city as sophisticated and efficiently run as your body, I'd want to live there.

Your body is constantly under attack from outside forces, and the skin is its greatest defender. It functions like Gore-tex, a high-tech outer sheath that protects us from temperature extremes, wind, and ultraviolet rays from the sun. It's a two-way barrier that not only retains water in the body but also acts as a water-resistant raincoat against too much water coming in. It's also our best shield against injury (bruises, cuts, and scrapes) and infection.

This incredible packaging contains us and keeps the body in balance by regulating temperature and providing insulation from heat and cold. For example, all the hair follicles are attached to tiny muscles that contract as a response to cold air, elevating hair on the body and trapping air around us, keeping the body warm like fur. When it's hot outside, cooling mechanisms kick into gear as the nervous system triggers the blood vessels and sweat glands to release heat as fast as possible. Overheated blood is pumped away from the heart and out to the skin, where the heat dissipates (which is why your skin becomes flushed). Sweating cools the skin by bringing moisture to the surface, where it evaporates in the air—instant air-conditioning.

As if all this weren't enough, the skin has the added role of synthesizing vitamin D, which is necessary for the absorption of bone-building calcium. The nutrient can also be obtained from milk and vitamin D–fortified juice and foods, as well as salmon, sardines, and fish oil. (Vitamin D supplements aren't easily absorbed into the system, so they don't work as effectively.) Luckily, a more palatable primary source of the vitamin is the sun. Vitamin D is known as "the sunshine vitamin" not because the sun has the nutrient in it but because UV rays actually convert a chemical found in the epidermis into vitamin D.

The Architecture of the Skin

There are three fundamental layers of the skin: the epidermis, the dermis, and the subcutaneous fat layer. There are four epidermal layers, the first of which is the stratum corneum. When you touch your skin, what you're feeling is almost thirty layers of dead keratin cells (a protein that also makes up hair and nails). All these inert cells, called keratinocytes, overlap like thin shingles on a roof, with pores (the ducts for hair follicles and sweat glands) interspersed among them. These tough keratinocytes shed approximately every twenty-eight days, depending on your skin's regenerative process. New cells that are formed in the lowest level of the epidermis push upward to the surface, constantly replacing the old ones. When your skin flakes, what's coming off are thousands of those dead cells. In fact, every minute we shed about forty thousand keratinocytes.

Just beneath the Gore-tex of the stratum corneum lies the brick wall of the epidermis. The "bricks" are squamous cells (durable keratinocytes that will eventually move up to the stratum corneum and be sloughed off) held together with rope-like bridges. The mortar is filled with fatty ceramides, which act as glue between the cells. Cells are "aquaphilic," meaning they allow water-soluble molecules to enter but won't let oil pass through them. Fatty ceramides are "lipophilic," allowing oil and fat substances to enter. This oil-and-water-don't-mix concept is one of the many barriers to substances (including most cosmetic ingredients) moving farther than this layer.

The first tier of the brick wall of the squamous cells is called the granular layer, where the soft keratin of the skin is made (as opposed to the hard keratin of nails and hair). Next is the spinous or squamous cell layer, the thick middle tier of the epidermis. Under that is the basal layer, where basal cells (which eventually become the keratinocytes on the skin's surface) generate. As the cells divide and mature, they move up, pushing older cells up to the surface, where they ultimately shed. When the basal cells reach the spinous layer, they are referred to as squamous cells. (In the skin, basal and squamous cells are both forms of keratinocytes; their names simply indicate where they are in the epidermis and in the cell maturation process.) As the keratinocytes reach the stratum corneum, they are cut off from the nourishment in the dermis and become a flatter, harder protein (keratin), until they die and flake off completely. This is the life cycle of the epidermis.

Beneath these elaborately woven levels of the epidermis lies the cement-like basement membrane, which glues the epidermis to the dermis. Lying under all those strata, the dermis seems as if it would be deeper down, but it's only one millimeter past the surface of your skin—less than the thickness of your thumbnail! But as you can see, getting there is no easy feat. Just imagine, this is the place all the cosmeceuticals are trying to reach, and they have to get through all those impressive, highly sophisticated tiers, not to mention the cement of the basement membrane, to get there. It's like trying to reach a castle behind obstacles like multiple barbed-wire fences, high brick walls, and moats full of killer crocodiles—a nearly impossible challenge. The dermis is where all the action is.

The dermis is where collagen and elastin are found, which is one reason it's the coveted destination for most of the active ingredients found in cosmetic products. In fact, the protein collagen makes up 70 percent of the dermis. It is a dense filler, much like the Styrofoam we use to pack fragile things. Elastin is connective tissue, the fine rubber bands, so to speak, that hold the foamy collagen in place so everything can flex and move. The beautiful scaffolds of collagen and elastin anchor the precious, vulnerable structures in the dermis in place and protect them from injury. Almost twice as thick as the epidermis above it, this rich layer is packed with nerve receptors that trigger sensation in our skin, blood vessels that transport oxygen and nutrients, sweat and oil glands, and hair follicles.

When we see pores on our skin, we're looking at either hair follicles or glands. The sebaceous, or oil, glands are attached to the hair follicles, which explains why the T-zone of the face, where hair follicles are the most dense, tends to get oily in most of us. The apocrine glands, which develop during puberty, are also attached to hair follicles in the genital area and the underarms and secrete sweat and body odor linked to sexual pheromones. Eccrine, or sweat, glands are spread out all over the body and help regulate temperature.

Just below the dermis is the aptly named subcutaneous fat layer, which covers the muscles. It provides shock-absorbent padding for the body and an insulating layer to conserve heat. The fat stored here also serves as an energy source. Coursing through this level are big ropes of collagen to keep the fatty tissue quilted in place and bigger blood vessels that feed the smaller vessels in the dermis above.

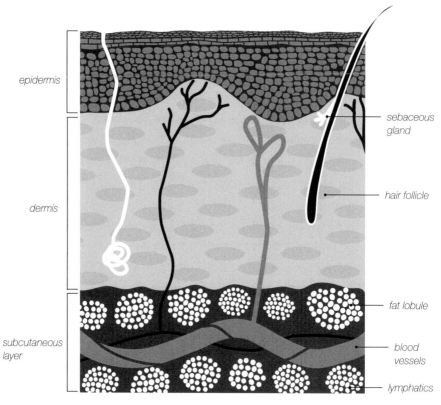

epidermis

dermis

subcutaneous
layer

sebaceous
gland

hair follicle

fat lobule

blood
vessels

lymphatics

A close-up picture of skin anatomy

The Action-Packed Work of Skin Cells

Like the bustling, invisible world of Who-ville, the universe of the skin
is inhabited by millions of microscopic workers—the cells. In biology
the concept of "structure is function" is vital, and it's exquisitely illus-
trated here. The entire body is built like a Lego set, with each piece
linking to others very specifically. Every cell's structure is designed for
a precise purpose. It's an efficient lock-and-key system in which a certain action in the body is unlocked, or activated, by one particular
kind of cell that has just the right key.

Melanocytes, for example, have the crucial job of producing melanin, the pigment that absorbs ultraviolet light from the sun. Ultraviolet

wavelengths can damage or destroy the DNA in cells, causing mutations that can turn into cancers. Once the skin is exposed to sunlight, the melanocytes try to cover all the cells with melanin, like sun hats that block UV rays. Ironically, though most of us feel that a suntan is a beautiful sign of health, it's actually a visible response to skin trauma, since the pigment has been produced to shield our cells' DNA from danger.

Sensing any kind of danger in the skin, the Langerhans cells, located in the epidermis and the dermis, are like the air traffic controllers of the immune system. They send out special agents—immune cells such as T cells and B cells—to capture foreign invaders such as bacteria and viruses, and fight off injuries like cuts and scrapes. They constantly monitor the environment of the skin for unsafe situations and send immune cells on their missions to bring back information about any trespasser. Then the body can decide to amass a great force of inflammatory cells to fight off the attacker by creating an allergic reaction or forming scar tissue.

Housed inside the hair follicle are stem cells, "pluripotential" cells that have the capacity to develop into any kind of cell they're needed to become. They can turn into collagen, skin, or immune cells if necessary, but once they have specialized they can't change again. Stem cells are similar to wild cards played in a game of poker, able to be converted into whatever incarnation will serve us best. In fact, scientists are now investigating the use of skin stem cells as an alternative to human embryonic stem cells in research that has the potential to cure illnesses such as Alzheimer's and Parkinson's and many different cancers. So the skin, this amazing and dynamic organ, will have latent possibilities in exciting medical research that promises to save lives in the future.

The fibroblast cells' extremely important function is to make collagen and elastin (the darlings of the cosmeceutical world). The skin's healing process is driven by these cells, which race to repair skin by making a scar or replenishing collagen to rebuild the structural integrity of the skin. It's probably no surprise to learn that as we age these cells get lazy and slow down production of this coveted protein. But we'll get to all the cold, hard facts about aging skin a bit later.

For now, ponder these numbers: the average square inch of skin (about the diameter of a quarter) can have approximately 65 hair follicles, 650 sweat glands, 20 blood vessels, more than a thousand nerve endings, and 60,000 melanocytes.

Our skin is a miniuniverse indeed, and one we should treat with quite a bit of wonder and complete consideration.

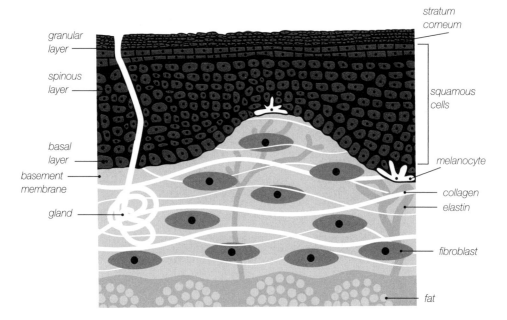

The intricate cellular architecture of the skin

2

There Are No Skin Types

My patients often ask me what kind of skin type they have. This stumps me almost every time. Of course, each of us tends to have a certain kind (whether it be dry, oily, or sensitive) most of the time. But skin is dynamic, changing in some way almost every day. Tying yourself down to one static "type" is less effective than being mindful of the changes in your skin and flexible in response. You need to learn how to read your skin and then tend to it using common sense. For instance, if your skin feels dry, apply a moisturizer. If your nose is particularly oily, use a degreaser such as salicylic acid on that specific area. Being attentive to your general tendency, or skin type, is a good first step in understanding how to treat your skin, but it's really just the beginning. Don't let it lock you in. It's more important to adjust your regimen for the type of skin you're having today—and to realize that it could be slightly different tomorrow.

Our complexions are a lot like our personalities: pretty unpredictable and influenced by our environments, both inside and out. Would you define yourself as always irritable or constantly bubbly and happy?

Of course not. We are complex creatures, with many different moods and facets to ourselves. Boiling it down to one or two unvarying traits is simply too restrictive. In a single day, hundreds of situations present themselves and will modify that persona. Someone cuts you off in traffic, and you become angry; your husband leaves his clothes on the floor again, and you're frustrated; your three-year-old gives you a hug, and all of a sudden you are joyful and content.

In the same way, a variety of factors can alter the skin's appearance each day. For instance, my complexion is usually sensitive and on the dry side. But today I'm breaking out around my mouth and chin. This could be due to my menstrual cycle, which, come to think of it, could also be making me moody too. This temporary condition doesn't mean I have acne or that I'm a sensitive person all of the time. Understanding what's going on in my world and my body can help me adjust my skin products, behaviors, or attitude to these changes.

Fitzpatrick Skin Types: Which One Are You?

From a doctor's perspective, the only real "skin type" classifications are Fitzpatrick Skin Types 1 to 6. Categorized by skin color, they gauge how a skin type responds to the sun. They may reflect ethnic variations in skin color as well. Type 1 is extremely fair and prone to sunburns, while Type 6 is very dark skin that rarely if ever burns. This scale assists a dermatologist in choosing the appropriate treatment for a patient. For example, one kind of laser may be safer for a particular skin type than another. Sure, a description such as "pale white skin that's usually sensitive" is pretty general, and each complexion is uniquely unpredictable and changeable. However, it's still a decent way to gauge how to treat it.

Even though most of us do not fit perfectly into a single rigid physical description, this classification system provides a general scale from lightest to darkest and corresponds to key problems that often crop up for each. In fact, feel free to put the word "usually" in front of the description and issues, as in "Type 1 usually has pale skin, light eyes, and blond or red hair, is usually Caucasian, and usually has redness and freckling." Most Asian women, for example, would be classified as a Type 2, with light skin and dark hair and eyes, and they usually have sensitive skin and hyperpigmentation issues.

FITZPATRICK SKIN TYPES

TYPE	COLOR	KEY SKIN ISSUES
1	Pale skin with light eyes and hair	Redness and freckling
2	Light skin with medium-dark hair and eyes	Sensitivity, redness, hyperpigmentation
3	Medium, olive, or golden skin and medium-dark hair and eyes	Hyperpigmentation
4	Deeper olive skin with dark hair and eyes	Sensitivity
5	Dark brown skin with dark hair and eyes	Hyperpigmentation
6	Black skin and hair, dark eyes	Hyperpigmentation, hypopigmentation (lightening of skin), keloids

Although terms such as "oily," "dry," "combination," and "sensitive" are more often linked to marketing campaigns than to medicine, they can also be very useful as troubleshooting clues. These generalizations are a springboard to a better awareness of how your skin reacts to external influences (the environment) and internal factors (a medication you are taking). So start by asking yourself, "Does my skin tend to be dry most of the time?" and "Do I usually have an oily T-zone?" But don't stop there. Being in tune with your skin and the rest of your body is as important as being in touch with your feelings, but most of us aren't paying enough attention to either one.

I'm amazed at the number of people who come into my office with dry skin all over their body and complain, "I'm so red and itchy. What's going on?" I ask, "Do you moisturize your skin?" and they say, "No." Problem solved. You'd be surprised how many people with chronically dry skin misdiagnose themselves with a skin disorder, when they simply need a moisturizer. Sometimes a prescription is just that simple, and you can be your own dermatologist by listening to your body. If your skin becomes red or gets irritated or stings when you put on any kind of moisturizer, it is being sensitive. In response, you can use products with anti-inflammatory ingredients such as aloe vera and soy. And stay away from irritating substances such as glycolic acid, chemical sunscreen, and certain preservatives and detergents. (I'll go into detail about the ingredients and skin routines in the following pages.)

In order to assess the condition of a patient's skin and get to the bottom of a problem, I ask a few questions. It's important to realize that skin does not exist in a vacuum. The way it reacts is tied to everything in your life. If you wake up and have pimples, you need to ask yourself, "Am I under stress?" "Did I eat something strange?" "Am I getting my period?" To evaluate what kind of skin you are having (and why), do some reconnaissance work and ask constructive questions of yourself. Once you solve the mystery of why your skin is behaving a certain way, you have a better chance of remedying it successfully.

Skin Evaluation Questions

▶ How does my skin usually behave? Does it tend to be dry or oily? Does it get irritated or red or hyperpigment easily? (A telltale sign of sensitivity.)

▶ What is my lifestyle like? Have I been doing anything differently in the last few weeks?

▶ What climate do I live in, or have I traveled somewhere recently? Is it a cold season with dry heaters in my home, or am I in a humid climate?

▶ What foods have I been eating lately?

▶ What kinds of products do I use on my skin and how often?

▶ What kind of makeup do I wear?

▶ How many showers a day do I take?

▶ Do I have a stressful job?

▶ Do I smoke?

▶ Do I take any medications regularly, even aspirin?

▶ Am I pregnant? Have I recently had a baby?

▶ Have I had surgery or any health problems in the last year?

▶ Do I wear sunscreen?

▶ Do I pick at my face nervously?

▶ How many products do I use on my skin and hair everyday?

▶ Do I touch my face a lot?

▶ Do I use hair gel or pomades?

▶ Is there a specific area on my face that is consistently a problem?

3

Factors That Influence Your Skin

We give the beauty of our skin incredibly high importance and consideration (in comparison to our blood pressure and other less noticeable facets of our bodies), but ironically, that importance is the inverse of the biological priority list. The body is most concerned with keeping the core—the heart and brain—in prime working order, so the skin is the low organ on the totem pole. Though it's one of the last priorities for the body, it is the first line of defense against exposure to cold, wind, and sun. So our selfless skin receives a battering from the outside and a certain amount of neglect from the inside. It deserves all the attention it can get. Because our skin is literally in our face, we can actually see how a host of influences impacts it all the time.

It's no wonder that we're so focused on the condition of our complexion, since it's the only body organ that we can evaluate in the mirror. That vanity is a very good thing. If our lungs or hearts were on display, making them appear healthy and beautiful would probably be a higher priority, and we'd all be in better shape. The bottom line: if wrinkles and premature aging scare you into wearing sunblock or quitting cigarettes, then bravo vanity!

I always tell my patients, "Take excellent care of your body, and I guarantee you'll look better too." Exercise and a healthy diet are good for your heart and the blood vessels that oxygenate the body, so they will ultimately benefit your skin too. Eating right, getting enough sleep, cutting down on stress—all these enable your systems to do their jobs. And a healthy complexion is part of the package. The antioxidants you eat and the eight hours of sleep you get may not go directly and immediately to your skin, but the trickle-down effect—along with other parts of your body—allows your skin to eventually reap the rewards.

Even though it may seem superficial, the state of your skin can actually tell you quite a lot. Sandwiched between the open air of the outside world and the internal body it protects, the skin reacts to both external ("extrinsic" in doctorspeak) and internal ("intrinsic") factors. Figuring out the reason behind a skin issue or tendency is the first step in improving your complexion. For example, a vacation in a dry climate may turn your skin into itchy, dehydrated sandpaper (eczema). Once you realize the "why" behind that dryness (the arid environment), you know the problem is temporary and can be easily remedied by using more moisturizer during your trip—or at worst, a steroid cream.

The reasons behind your skin's behavior provide not only clues to a prescription but a way to prevent a problem from happening. If you learn that using a certain type of topical ingredient or eating a particular kind of food exacerbates a condition, you can avoid it. For instance, eating spicy food and drinking alcohol tend to make rosacea worse. If that happens to be the case for you, managing the problem is clear: an ounce of prevention is worth a pound of cure.

The "why" can also be profoundly insightful, because the skin is a magnifying glass into the body. If an illness is causing a reaction on the skin, catching it early not only relieves the initial problem, it can sometimes provide a more profound solution. For example, it's common for women who come in for acne treatments to have a little extra hair on certain parts of the body, and these two things can be symptoms of polycystic ovarian syndrome. Dermatologists are trained to read the skin for small, classic signs that diagnose other, larger health problems.

Undoubtedly, some of the factors I'll discuss in the following pages can be considered both internal *and* external. The external stress of being stuck in traffic every day or having your boss yell at you may seem initially to hit you from the outside. But if you think about it from the perspective of your skin, it is affected by how the nervous system *inside* your body reacts to that outside stress. What you eat and drink comes from outside your body as well, but your skin reacts to the nutrients (or the chemicals, spices, or fats) from the inside out. Regardless of the ins and outs of these various influences, they can cause the skin to react in both positive and negative ways. All these "whys" play a part in how your complexion behaves, and they will help you be a great diagnostician when reading your own skin.

Internal Factors

Heredity and Your Ethnic Background

Family history is the biggest intrinsic influence on the kind of skin you have. Genetics have everything to do with your skin's tendency toward dryness, oiliness, or sensitivity. A person inherits conditions such as psoriasis, acne, eczema, rosacea, and even a predisposition to skin cancers (which is tied to skin color). Genetics is the way your DNA deck has been shuffled. So if you have fair skin that tends to get red easily and is very sensitive, it's more than likely that your mother, father, or grandparents handed down that trait. Certainly, sensitive skin can be both generated or exacerbated by other factors (such as the use of irritating skin products), but you were also probably dealt a sensitive skin card in that DNA deck.

Heredity and ethnicity are obviously related (pardon the pun), and the skin color passed down from your parents plays an especially important role in your skin's relationship to the sun and to other factors as well. In the last chapter, I discussed Fitzpatrick Skin Types, a classification system devised in 1975 by a dermatologist, Thomas B. Fitzpatrick, MD, PhD, of Harvard Medical School. Types 1 to 6 are categorized by skin color and based on how each responds to UV rays. Dermatologists use this scale to gauge what kind of laser or light treatment is appropriate and safe for a particular skin type or color.

Type 1s, like me, have pale skin with light eyes and tend to burn easily. They are prone to skin sensitivity and rosacea and, of course, sunburn. Because of this, they may be more predisposed to skin cancers such as melanoma. Asian skin is usually a Type 2 or 3 and has a propensity for producing brown patches, or melasma. Types 4 and 5 tend to be of Hispanic, African-American or Asian ethnicities, and are often more prone to hyperpigmentation, as is Type 6. Type 6s have very dark skin, and because they have more melanin, they almost never burn in the sun. (Remember that melanocytes produce melanin to absorb ultraviolet rays.) That increased melanin offers Type 6s more natural sun protection but also increases their tendency to hyperpigmentation. A tiny acne scar can become a dark brown stain, for example. So skin color and family history are important players in how your skin behaves from the very beginning.

Health, Illness, and Medications

A healthy body is going to maintain a healthy complexion, along with all the other amazing functions in your system. On the flip side, when the body is weak, it cannot nourish the skin well. (The skin is low on the totem pole, remember?) Illness forces the immune system to work overtime to fix what's wrong, and the skin takes a backseat. Skin provides an X-ray vision into what's going on in your body. If you're sick, your skin is going to show it. Itchy, dry skin, especially on the lower legs, can be the first indication of diabetes. Even a fungal infection such as athlete's foot can be a warning sign, as are cold skin in the extremities, white patches of skin (vitiligo), and poor wound healing. On the other hand, when internal illness manifests itself on the surface of your body, there's good news: you might be able to catch the disease that's causing it early.

>>> A REAL PATIENT STORY:
Dermatology Is Detective Work

I believe that a podiatrist or a manicurist who's on the ball can catch symptoms of a serious health problem, because the nails offer telltale signs of internal trouble. I can actually read someone's health history right on the nails. I was examining a patient recently, and when I got to her nails, I asked, "Do you have iron-deficiency anemia?" She said, "Yes." Then I asked if she'd stopped taking her iron supplements about three months before, and she answered affirmatively, wondering how I could possibly know that. I knew because she had koilonychia, concave, spoon-shaped nails. Since hers was on the middle of her nail (and the growth cycle of fingernails is six months), I could tell the approximate time period since she had stopped taking her supplements. I suggested that she start taking her supplements again and the concave indentation would grow out eventually. Anything traumatic can affect nails' growth cycle (the same goes for the skin and hair, but it's less obvious). If you get a really bad flu or a fever, three to six months later you may notice a white horizontal band or indentation on some of your nails. It's called a Beau's line, and indicates that the nails stopped growing during a period of physical or emotional stress. Another patient's lunulas, the white half-moons near the cuticle, went all the way up to the middle of the nails. When I saw this, I checked the patient's blood work because it could have meant that he had kidney problems related to diabetes or other diseases. The shape of the nails is just as informative. Some people have clubbing, and the tips of the nails are curved and slightly bulbous. This usually occurs in patients who have congestive heart failure or smoke too much (because not enough oxygen is reaching the tips of their fingers). It's almost a form of a scar. The clubbing may go away if the patient stops smoking or improves the condition of his or her heart.

The nails' color can be just as informative as their shape. One patient came in with a light blue-gray discoloration of all of his nails. That led me to ask him questions about his family history, because it could have indicated either a collagen vascular disease or some kind of drug toxicity or hypersensitivity. It turned out he was taking the antibiotic minocycline, and it had caused a reaction. I recommended that he stop taking that medication. When I examine a patient, I take a look at everything from head to toe. The skin is an atlas to what's going on inside the rest of the body, and even the fingernails can relay valuable information.

The prescription and nonprescription drugs we take can be the cause of many skin conditions, from chronic dryness to bruising or rashes. Many people who take an aspirin every day to lower their risk of heart attack or stroke get bruises all over the body because their blood doesn't clot well. If I'm doing a skin check and notice a lot of bruising, especially on bony areas, I ask if the patient is taking aspirin, Aleve, ibuprofen, or Plavix every day. They're usually on too much blood thinner, which causes any little bump to the body to leave a bruise. The vessels near the surface of the skin show me that the rest of the body is at risk for trauma too. The herbal supplement Saint John's wort (taken as an antidepressant) can also thin the blood, as can garlic, vitamin E, and gingko biloba. (For this reason, I always advise patients to stop taking any of these before having surgery or an injectable cosmetic procedure.) Lithium, a drug used to treat both epilepsy and bipolar disorder, can cause horrendous acne and chronic folliculitis, and it can exacerbate psoriasis. Anyone taking a sulfur medication such as Bactrim (a common medication for urinary tract infections) can develop extreme photosensitivity reactions in the sunlight. Sometimes a patient displays a red rash that mimics eczema but is actually an allergic drug reaction to some kind of medicine. Some people get recurrent red circles, always in the same place on the body. This bizarre rash comes and goes. It can be a fixed drug reaction or eruption related to smoking marijuana or to taking tetracycline antibiotics or even ibuprofen. (I suppose that Advil excuse could come in handy for some people?)

>>> A REAL PATIENT STORY:
Skin Problems Can Be Side Effects of Medication

Frequently very good medications that generate positive results for the body can create negative reactions in the skin. A man came into my office complaining of terribly chapped, cracked lips. They were painful to the point where he was having trouble eating. He'd been to different doctors and had been given different medicines to treat his cheilitis, the medical term for inflammation of the lips (one manifestation of the condition is dryness, cracking, and chapping). But because the cause of his chapped lips was unknown, these medications were just temporary Band-Aids. The patient also showed me two eczema-like rashes on his ankles (lichen simplex chronicus), which looked and felt like alligator skin. I asked what medications he was taking, then went back through the time line of when his lips had started to bother him. Everything was linked very closely to Lipitor, the statin drug used to control high cholesterol, which was drying out his skin to this extreme. Piecing together a time line is tricky, because in general it takes about two weeks to have a reaction to a new medication, but you could also have a delayed reaction much later on. The prescription is just as problematic: he could have considered discontinuing the Lipitor, but one of the side effects of all statin drugs is dry skin. The immediate cure was to treat his dry skin symptoms. I treated him with a simple emollient cream and a short course of a steroid ointment. I also advised him to speak to his internist about alternatives to statins.

>>> q&a

Q: My friend was recently diagnosed with breast cancer. After surgery, she's undergoing chemotherapy and radiation. I've heard that these treatments can cause extreme skin irritation, like a blistering rash, is this true?

A: Unfortunately the side effects of many cancer treatments add insult to injury—especially since the body's immune system is so compromised. I realize that a rash or other skin irritations seem low on the list of your friend's worries, but they can be severely uncomfortable and sometimes can even be life threatening. Most require the attention of a doctor since they are associated with crucial medical treatment, and even mild reactions should be reported to the oncologist at once. This is not a simple, irritating rash, and your friend absolutely should not suffer in silence or try to treat it herself.

The issue of drug reactions that occur on the skin is extremely important (it can affect the course of treatment), and the problem is actually quite complex. There are dermatologists who specialize solely in this area. In fact, it's wise for anyone preparing to go through radiation or chemotherapy to ask their oncologist to recommend a dermatologist who specializes in drug reactions. There are as many variations of skin side effects (rashes, inflammation, blistering, itching) as there are cancer treatments, and even though some medicines have classic rashes—on hands and feet—each individual patient may react uniquely. When I was doing my training at Memorial Sloan-Kettering Cancer Center in New York, I saw many different types of chemotherapy and radiation dermatitis every day, in all kinds of cancer patients. Since some patients were taking fifteen different medications, the crucial question was: which drug is causing the reaction, and will the rash progress to a more critical level? If so, the dose of medication or radiation may be reduced, or sometimes stopped.

Drug eruptions are often characteristic of certain medications. For example, targeted chemotherapy drugs (that zone in on one area of the body)—such as Taxol, for breast cancer—can cause fingernails and cuticles to become swollen and inflamed (a nail disease called paronychia). Taxol can also trigger an acne-like rash on the face, which should *not* be treated as acne. It actually needs to be cared for with moisturizer. Side effects like these occur because a targeted therapy uses chemicals that react with cancer cells, but can have a cross reaction with receptors on other cells too (like those on the skin). Regular chemotherapy—which essentially uses toxic chemicals to kill cancer cells—can also affect normal, healthy cells and cause a host of hypersensitivity reactions, such as hair loss, severe itching, swelling, dry skin and an increased bruising. It's sensible to consult the oncologist before taking anything like an antihistamine for itching or vitamin K for bruising, since even over-the-counter medications and supplements can react negatively with other medications being taken.

During radiation, almost every patient can expect some kind of rash within a few days or weeks after beginning treatment. Since radiation is localized, the side effects are usually confined to the "field of radiation." Acute reactions make the skin red and inflamed. Sometimes it can appear sunburned or tan (inflammatory hyperpigmentation), or it can become a blistering rash. You can lose hair in the area, or skin can become scaly and dry. Other side effects may be dry mouth and lips, sore gums and inflammation of the mucous membranes. Acute radiation dermatitis has a direct relationship to the dose of radiation a patient is receiving. It may be necessary to reduce that amount, so it's vital to inform the radiation oncologist of any skin symptoms (even something mild, like redness). For short term relief, I usually recommend using a rich emollient (like Aquaphor) for dry, reddened skin. Avoid any products with drying irritants like fragrance or alcohol and be especially careful about sun protection (since this vulnerable skin is hypersensitive to the sun). The good news is that there are many effective OTC products specifically made for chemo and radiation rashes. One is Lindi Skin Cooler Pads (www.lindiskin.com) with aloe and green tea to soothe the inflamed area. Products like this can be found online, but consult your physician first to be on the safe side. The oncologist may have a few good suggestions too.

Chronic, long-term effects of radiation can appear even six months after treatment. A patient may notice thickened, scar-like skin in the area, which can be extremely uncomfortable and difficult to treat. As with acute chemotherapy and radiation rashes, a dermatologist will often prescribe topical steroids to treat these side effects.

Obviously this is a very complicated and difficult topic, but in general, it's important to remember the basic principles of skin care (such as applying an emollient ointment to moisturize and protect a dry, irritated area), and it is essential that patients communicate clearly with their medical team. Your friend must report any information about side effects from medication or treatment. She should not consider this complaining or whining. It is useful information that will help the doctor do a more effective job.

Hormones

There are multitudes of different hormones in your body. They act as chemical messengers, carrying specific signals from one cell to another and regulating the function of their target cells. Hormones beautifully exemplify the biological lock-and-key concept of "structure is function," in that each particular hormone has a key to a receptor on (or inside) a specific type of cell. This complex communication system can also have many different effects on your complexion. Hormones are supposed to be in balance, but often they surge or dip, wreaking havoc on the skin.

The sex hormones—estrogen, progesterone, and testosterone—take a lot of blame when it comes to problem skin, especially acne flare-ups. During puberty there's a huge surge of hormones that cause growth and development. Remember that the sebaceous glands are attached to the hair follicles; these kick into action during this amazing growth spurt. Male hormones called "androgens" (found in males and

females) trigger these glands to produce more oil, and if the hair follicles become clogged with dead skin cells, the oil doesn't have a way to
get out. The unfortunate result is acne.

For the same hormonal reasons, the menstrual cycle is a surefire
trigger for regular breakouts. Estrogen and progesterone levels spike at
different times during the cycle, and when the androgenic progesterone rises (just before ovulation) it activates the sebaceous glands,
which in turn causes premenstrual acne. This yin and yang of estrogen
and progesterone is why acne develops, so taking birth control pills,
which keep the hormones at a more consistent level, seems to keep
breakouts at bay. Because the surges of androgens aren't so severe,
there tend to be fewer flare-ups linked to them.

Wildly fluctuating hormones during pregnancy can create an awful
complexion or a radiant glow, often in the same woman. For the first
twelve weeks, the growth hormone human chorionic gonadotropin
(HCG) surges to prepare the placenta and increase the blood volume
in the body. (This can create a flushed, healthy complexion as the
blood flow becomes more robust.) In the second trimester, progesterone is on the upswing, which can generate acne. Another possible, and
common, consequence of increased progesterone and estrogen is
melasma, a brown discoloration above the upper lip and on the cheeks
and forehead, which is why it's known as "the mask of pregnancy." On
the other hand, many women find that their complexion remains clear
and their skin tone is beautiful during their entire pregnancy. It really
is the luck of the draw when it comes to unpredictable hormones, and
every woman's skin will display different reactions. (I had terrible
melasma—it's really distressing.)

As a woman begins to go through menopause, her hormone
levels begin a steep drop-off. Sweating through hot flashes and dryness are the top skin complaints during this time, because estrogen
and progesterone aren't telling the sebaceous glands to pump out as
much oil. Lower levels of these hormones also diminish angiogenesis, or the growth of new blood vessels, which can also contribute to

a dull complexion. These intense hormone imbalances can also trigger dilation of the blood vessels on the surface of the skin, which creates a spike in temperature and temporarily flushed and clammy skin (otherwise known as a "hot flash"). It's similar to a stress response surge of blood to the surface of the skin. Basically, the communication of some of these hormonal messengers has slowed to a crawl, so many of their functions aren't sparked off. Science has proven that declining estrogen levels are associated with skin changes such as dryness, poor wound healing, decreased skin laxity and collagen content, and epidermal thinning and increased transepidermal water loss (diminished moisture on the surface of the skin).[1] Medical studies are evaluating the effects of hormone replacement therapy (HRT) on these skin changes, and some results show that HRT (which provides a low dose of estrogen and progesterone) increases sebum secretion and seems to be associated with beneficial effects on skin collagen levels and skin thickness.[2] Estrogen also appears to increase mucopolysaccharide and hyaluronic acid levels in the skin, which maintain skin hydration.[3]

Although HRT may be helpful for some, it's still a controversial solution for many of us. It's indicated only if you are symptomatic, meaning suffering from bone loss or severe hot flashes or dry skin. And it's definitely a subject to discuss with your doctor.

The ups and downs of hormones aren't all about the reproductive system. There are all kinds of hormones in the body, and they can indirectly impact the skin too. Low thyroid hormone (hypothyroidism) causes fish scale–like thickening of the skin that's rough and dry (myxedema). The skin on the hands and feet can turn yellow, the hair on the eyebrows can fall out, other hair becomes coarse, and brittle, and the nails break easily. Hyperthyroidism, caused by too much thyroid hormone, creates the opposite reaction in the skin: it may become moist and smooth, with a tendency to flush and get red. Some people with hyperthyroidism get a bronzed appearance to the skin (melanoderma) and even melasma on the cheeks. All these different hormonal messengers have the potential to get out of balance and when they get their wires crossed, the skin can definitely show it.

What You Eat and Drink

Doesn't it seem that every time you pick up a magazine there's another article on some superfood that's going to make your skin healthy and gorgeous? (Acai is the new pomegranate, and goji berry is the new blueberry!) Who can keep it all straight? And, honestly, who needs to? Most of the information I read about nutrition for the skin centers on eating nourishing fruits, vegetables, fish, and whole grains—a balanced diet, basically, that will impact your complexion in a positive way. And it will—in the same way that most of these other intrinsic factors, such as medications you take, influence it—indirectly. After all, eating a healthy diet is beneficial for *all* of you, not just your face. Again, we place so much importance on our skin, but it reflects what's going on in the whole body.

The food you put into your mouth has an effect once it's been metabolized and delivered to the skin. The way it's metabolized is also why eating certain foods, though beneficial to both the skin and body, may not affect the complexion directly. The body breaks down what we eat into tiny particles of proteins, fats, and carbohydrates. Food is circulated in its smallest form, so that nutrients can be reconstructed and repackaged, and then transported to the organs that need them. Eventually nutrients get to the skin too. (Remember that the skin doesn't take precedence in the body.) It's like a factory conveyor belt with lots of things happening at once, so it's not realistic to imagine that eating an avocado or a piece of salmon will deliver healthy fatty acids straight to your skin. That being said, it's a good idea to incorporate skin-healthy foods into your diet, especially olive oil, avocados, salmon, sunflower seeds, Brazil nuts, wheat germ, broccoli, and leafy greens.

The body is constantly under construction, but instead of hammers and nails it uses chemical reactions and vitamins and nutrients from food to repair and rebuild. My bottom line? Keep it simple, and stick to the basics. Eat a balanced diet of good-for-you foods—including fruits, vegetables, healthy fats, whole grains, dairy, lean meat, and fish. Eating healthfully should supply your body (and ultimately your skin) with the building blocks they need. Avoid prepared foods. Try olives, sunflower seeds, or fruit instead of addictive, salty chips or bogus energy bars.

As popular as the "super skin foods" topic may be in magazines, there's not much sound scientific evidence behind all of it yet. Scientists are studying the effects of many foods and vitamins on the health of the skin, but strong studies are still pretty scarce. Even so, there are things you can eat that definitely benefit the skin in particular, and deficiencies of certain nutrients is damaging. A lack of protein can lead to poor wound healing and hair loss, and a fat deficiency can bring on dry skin and brittle hair and nails. A lack of vitamin C can cause scurvy (yes, even in this day and age!), which leads to spongy gums and bleeding hair follicles, among other awful skin conditions. So don't be caught short of the nutrients your skin needs in your diet, but don't make yourself crazy either. It's really not too difficult to incorporate essential food elements into your daily meals.

Top Substances in Food That Optimize Skin Health

>>> VITAMINS C AND E

Vitamin C is found in: Oranges, lemons, grapefruit, papaya, and tomatoes

Vitamin E is found in: Sweet potatoes, nuts, olive oil, sunflower seeds, avocados, broccoli, and leafy green vegetables

What they do for skin: These antioxidant vitamins fight oxidation damage in skin cells' DNA. Because they are key elements in the structural proteins in the body, they are important to the integrity of the blood vessels and hair follicles. They're required for the formation of collagen, and medical studies have found that they decrease wrinkling of the skin.[4] Vitamin E reduces inflammation and helps wound healing. Vitamin C enhances the immune response.

>>> VITAMIN A

It's found in: Fish oil, salmon, carrots, dairy products, spinach, and broccoli

What it does for skin: Since it promotes normal keratinization (the turnover of skin cells), it helps with conditions such as acne, eczema, and psoriasis. Without it, skin becomes extremely dry and dull. It's important to note that if you use a synthetic retinoid (a derivative of vitamin A) on your skin, you may need to stop vitamin A supplementation, since too much of this vitamin can lead to hair loss and liver dysfunction.

>>> PROTEIN

It's found in: Meat, eggs, grains, sunflower seeds, dairy products, fish, legumes like beans and peas, and nuts such as walnuts and pecans

What it does for skin: Protein is a component of all the cells in the body and a building block of skin tissue. Proteins are broken down into amino acids, the building blocks of new proteins for the body's constant reconstruction job. They are like Legos, coming in different shapes, sizes, and types that help construct collagen or create lubricating ceramide in the skin. It's a perfect economy, with the amino acids being recycled into new proteins on a supply-and-demand basis.

>>> ZINC

It's found in: Turkey, almonds, Brazil nuts, and wheat germ

What it does for skin: This anti-inflammatory mineral calms irritation in the epidermis and helps to heal acne and treat rosacea. It also facilitates cell regeneration.

>>> BIOTIN

It's found in: Egg yolks, brewer's yeast, bananas, lentils, cauliflower, and salmon

What it does for skin: This B vitamin strengthens skin, hair, and nails. (A deficiency is extremely rare because bacteria in your intestines make all the biotin you need.) A deficit can lead to hair loss or dermatitis (itchy, scaly skin). Some people swear by biotin supplements to strengthen brittle nails, but studies haven't proven that it's beneficial for anyone who's not deficient in the vitamin.

>>> OMEGA-3 AND OMEGA-6 FATTY ACIDS

Omega-6 is found in: Seeds, nuts, eggs, and sunflower and soybean oil (which are in lots of snack foods, such as crackers, cookies, and cereals)

Omega-3 is found in: Cold-water fish such as salmon and sardines, flax-seed oil, walnuts, sunflower seeds, and almonds

What they do for skin: These essential fatty acids support skin health, improve nerve and vascular function, and act as antioxidants. Omega-3 has strong anti-inflammatory properties and may calm skin conditions such as rosacea or eczema and minimize redness. It also boosts immune system functioning. Some nutritional studies have shown that omega-3 may protect against squamous cell skin cancers and decrease sunburn response. Studies have shown that diets rich in the omega-6 fatty acid linoleic acid are associated with less skin dryness and thinning. But it's important to note that these fatty acids must be balanced in the body. For example, too much omega-6 and linoleic acid can cause an inflammatory response in the body, while omega-3 minimizes it. Because of the prevalence of omega-6 in processed snack foods, it's believed that we are getting an abundance of them and not enough omega-3. And studies have shown that too much omega-6 can increase the risk of everything from high blood pressure to dementia and depression. The key is balancing your intake of the two.

>>> MONOUNSATURATED FATS

They're found in: Olive oil, canola oil, and avocados

What they do for skin: These healthy fats help to maintain the water level in the epidermis and supply the ceramides and fats that keep the bricks and mortar of the skin healthy and intact. This translates into less itchy, healthy-looking, glowing skin.

>>> ANTIOXIDANTS

They're found in: Blueberries, green tea, red kidney beans, olive oil, artichokes, pomegranates, dark chocolate, and red wine

What they do for skin: These are indeed the superheroes of the nutrient family. We've heard a lot about how antioxidants extinguish the dangerous free radicals (the toxic oxygen molecules that can be by-products of cell renewal and are also generated by pollution and sun damage). The polyphenol antioxidants in green tea have also been shown to help prevent certain skin cancers and protect skin against sunburns. Antioxidants found in red wine and green tea are being studied for their possible cancer-fighting potential, but so far the results aren't conclusive. There have been studies that strongly showed that the antioxidants in green tea (among them epigallocatechin-3-gallate, or EGCG) protect the DNA in skin cells from UV-induced damage.[5]

Later, I will go into more detail about antioxidants (used topically and internally) and the booming trend of "nutriceutical" skin supplements, but my best advice in general is moderation. Ingesting too much of a good thing can be unproductive and possibly destructive. If you overconsume vitamin C, your system's protective mechanism expels the excess through urine, and ingesting too many vitamin supplements can have many potentially toxic effects. For instance, an overload of carotene (the type of vitamin A found in carrots) literally causes skin to turn orange and can lead to liver problems. Consider herbal and vitamin supplements to be drugs, and treat them with the same kind of cautious respect. It's wise to check with your doctor before embarking on any kind of supplementation program, and it's a good idea to check the USDA Recommended Dietary Allowance to see how much is too much. Keep in mind that the body absorbs and utilizes vitamins in food more effectively and efficiently than it digests supplements. Coming back to the body's amazing protective mechanism, it takes in only about 15 percent of the nutrient in a supplement if you don't have a deficiency, and the rest is excreted in urine.

We know there are foods that benefit the skin. There are also quite a few that can worsen some conditions. Once again, the jury is still out science-wise on the role of diet in skin health and disease. Many studies are inconclusive, and many are yet to be done. Nonetheless, some foods have been proven to make symptoms worse. Studies have shown that spicy foods and alcohol usually aggravate rosacea. Foods such as milk, eggs, soy, peanuts, and wheat have been known to make eczema worse. And though non-nutritious foods won't actually *cause* acne, there are some that may make it worse (check out the Q&A on the following page). A diet loaded with carbohydrates and sugar can cause flare-ups. If you have a skin issue that might be irritated by your diet, keep track of what you eat in a food journal. It will soon be apparent what triggers you need to avoid in the future.

A hot topic right now in the skin care world (and by that I mean the cosmetic more than the medical arena) is "glycation"—essentially, the idea that glucose (from carbohydrates and sugars) that you digest may attach to proteins such as collagen in your body and form new molecules called advanced glycation end products, or AGEs. These AGEs allegedly degrade collagen and elastin, causing them to harden and lose elasticity in the same way rust weakens and degrades metal. It's important to know that so far the only testing done on glycation and the skin has been in vitro (in a Petri dish in a laboratory), so there's a long way to go before it's proven that eating carbohydrates and sugars can destroy the collagen in the dermis. The current hype about glycation stems from solid scientific research that's been done about plaque buildup in the arteries and blood vessels of diabetics (who are unable to process sugars normally) and how this can lead to heart attacks and strokes. Glycation, which occurs when insulin doesn't metabolize sugars properly, destroys the collagen in blood vessels (collagen is a structural protein found all over the body, not just in the skin) and ultimately causes it to become brittle and form plaque. Can sugars do equally damaging things to collagen in the skin, even in people who don't suffer from diabetes? It's a very interesting theoretical question and a strong argument could be made, but there are as yet no human controlled studies to show the relevance of glycation to the skin. My suggestion to you: stick with a healthy, balanced diet. If you want a blueberry muffin, go ahead. Just don't eat them every day to the exclusion of other foods. Again, use logic and let moderation be your guide.

>>> q&a

Q: Does indulging in chocolate, junk food, and fatty meals cause acne?

A: The link between nutrition and acne is still controversial, and many medical studies are still to be done on the subject. But this much is scientifically proven: chocolate has gotten a bad rap as the instigator of pimple production. It has been proven that chocolate does not cause or aggravate the condition. The consequences of eating lots of junk food are less clear. Quite a few studies have shown that eating high-fat diets can increase sebaceous output.[6] Other research has found that dairy products set off acne (perhaps by triggering testosterone to activate the sebaceous glands).[7] A recent study published in the *Journal of the American Academy of Dermatology* found that adolescent boys with acne who ate a diet high in carbohydrates and processed foods showed no improvement in their complexions. The boys put on a healthy diet showed a substantial clearing of their acne. (The bonus: the high-protein, low-glycemic group also lost weight.)[8] Apparently, high-glycemic-index carbohydrates (stuff like pizza and cookies that are quickly converted into glucose) raise the blood sugar level, followed by a release of insulin and androgen hormones (the ones that signal the sebaceous glands to go for broke).

So it may make sense to stay away from dairy products such as milk and ice cream, as well as processed foods with a high carbohydrate and sugar content. Sounds like a teenager's worst nightmare. And although eating chocolate has not been scientifically proven to cause acne, I'm living proof that it does, so my bet is that science may actually find a link! Again, eating in moderation is the key—if it's possible with chocolate.

Q: Will drinking a lot of water make my skin look better?

A: Water has always been thought to provide benefits for the skin, but drinking huge amounts of it isn't going to make you look even better. The body will simply eliminate the excess through urination. However, water intoxication is a real, although uncommon condition, and it can kill you. It causes cells and tissue to swell to the point of bursting. It's also associated with electrolyte disturbance and hyponatremia, a dilution of sodium in the bloodstream. (Healthy kidneys can process fifteen liters of water per day, so unless your water intake is enormous, I wouldn't worry too much about a fatal water overdose.) The recommended amount is eight eight-ounce glasses a day, but if you exercise a lot you may need more, and for some people four glasses is sufficient. Twenty percent of our water intake comes from food (such as juicy fruits and vegetables), and that counts toward our daily drinking dose. But since the body conserves water for the more important organs (not the skin, as we know), what we ingest is utilized first by the heart, brain, liver, and kidneys before the skin gets a sip. So it is likely that most of us aren't drinking enough.

Water is essential to the skin's metabolism and regeneration (actions such as producing new skin cells and growing new hair in follicles). The highways bringing nutrients to your skin and taking metabolic debris away are the blood vessels. Water moves blood flow along smoothly and washes away toxic by-products (enzymes, amino acids, salts) from chemical reactions. The visible brightening effect that you see on your skin has to do with that robust circulation. It also increases the extracellular water in your facial tissues, so you may get a slight plumping effect. But refuting these facts, researchers at the University of Pennsylvania recently found no clinical evidence that water consumption is essential to helping the kidneys filter toxins more efficiently. Their findings also included this: drinking water can't actually hydrate the skin from the inside out. With all this contradictory information, how much water do you need to benefit the skin? Since the liquid you drink won't reach the stratum corneum, you're better off alleviating dry skin topically with a moisturizer that prevents water loss from the surface. Even though there may be no direct correlation between drinking water and plumping or moisturizing your skin, sufficient hydration is essential to keeping the body—and the skin—healthy. Ultimately, adequate water consumption (this means not drinking to excess but avoiding dehydration) is like eating a balanced diet: it's good for your body as a whole, your complexion included. Plus, water is essential to breaking down fat and losing weight.

Q: Does exercise or weight have any influence on my skin?

A: Being over- or underweight has negative effects on the body overall but doesn't have a huge influence on skin unless the loss or gain is extreme. Obesity, for example, puts a great deal of stress on the entire body and leads to swelling and skin breakdown. Researchers at Harvard University recently found that overweight women are at higher risk of developing psoriasis, an inflammatory skin disease. Women who had gained thirty-five pounds or more since the age of eighteen had an 88 percent greater risk for psoriasis than those whose weight had remained stable.[9] The study showed that fat deposits can lead to chronic, low-grade inflammation that may trigger the disease. Meanwhile, researchers at the University of Texas M. D. Anderson Cancer Center found that a restricted-calorie diet inhibits skin cancer (namely melanoma) in mice, while obesity triggers it by activating cell surface receptors that encourage the growth of many human cancers. It follows that losing weight, which is healthy in any case, may reduce the symptoms of psoriasis and decrease your risk of cancer. However, being underweight isn't good for your body, or your skin, either. A healthy, happy medium is key. Simple, right?

Exercise is great for your circulation, the conveyor belt that replenishes everything your skin needs, including the oxygen and nutrients that feed the cells. The rosy flush you get when you work out is a sign that your heart is pumping and providing better blood flow to the skin. Exercise also causes perspiration, which excretes salts and toxins through the skin, helping to keep it clear and acne-free. And it reduces stress, which in turn tends to quiet the adrenal glands and control the production of the androgen hormones that trigger acne.

Sleep (or the Lack of It)

Sleep deprivation is a form of stress that has become a national epidemic, which is no surprise. According to the National Commission on Sleep Disorder Research, approximately 70 million people in the United States are affected by a sleep problem. The National Institute of Health reports that 40 percent of American adults occasionally have difficulty sleeping, and more than half that number are women. A 2005 poll by the National Sleep Foundation found that women are more likely to experience sleep problems than men. This makes sense, considering we are usually the child-rearing caregivers in the family. On top of that, we're hormonally programmed to have sleeping issues. During pregnancy, nearly 80 percent of women have sleep disturbances, and during menopause an equal percentage suffer from interrupted sleep (thanks primarily to hot flashes).

So what does all this bad news have to do with our skin? Simply put, if you sleep too little, you're not giving the body time to repair itself. The nervous system has two states that are in balance. The sympathetic system, which is more in control while we're awake, keeps the blood flow near the core of the body. While we sleep, the parasympathetic nervous system runs the show and blood flow shifts to the skin. Additionally, skin isn't under attack from the sun and the elements at night. This relaxed parasympathetic state allows greater circulation and oxygen flow to the skin, or peripheral vasodilation in medical terms. This is when the skin gets a lot of internal attention and repair mechanisms go into action, much like the night workmen at Disneyland who fix and restore the rides and clean the place up before the park opens the next day. Receptors spring to life within the blood vessels and grab amino acid molecules (the building blocks) to help build more collagen, and fluid and toxins are drained.

Without enough rest, the skin doesn't get this repair and restoration, and all that important activity isn't being done. One example: when excess fluid near the skin isn't transported to the bladder to be excreted, the result is puffiness. (The kidneys work more actively during the parasympathetic state to convey excess fluid from the circulatory system to the bladder.) It shows up most around the eyes because there's less fat in that area, so water retention is more apparent. As far as dark circles go, a lack of sleep doesn't cause them (they have more to do with your anatomy, as you'll see in "Problems and Prescriptions" on page 215) but accentuates them because your skin appears dull and translucent (due to that lack of blood flow to the skin). A lot of research has examined how chronic sleep deprivation compromises the immune system. One study found that sleep deprivation disrupted women's skin barrier function (how the stratum corneum prevents water loss and blocks the entry to foreign substances), and this could trigger or exacerbate inflammatory disorders such as psoriasis, eczema, and atopic dermatitis.[10] All are reasons enough to get the seven to eight hours of recommended shut-eye you need per night.

Stress

Sleep deprivation is just one form of stress, which is a demand on your body that calls on it to do something. For example, if you eat too much food, your body has to work harder to digest it. Other forms of stress are illness, trauma, emotional distress, and pain. In order to cope, the nervous system's sympathetic "fight-or-flight" mechanism goes into overdrive to conserve energy at the core and protect the heart and brain. This puts the skin into a weakened state. It also releases hormones such as adrenaline and cortisol, which increase the heart rate, raise blood pressure and blood sugar levels, and suppress the immune system. Many studies have proven that chronic psychological stress stifles the immune system and impairs the epidermal barrier, which can delay wound healing and generate or aggravate skin disorders such as eczema. (Oddly enough, acute—very short-term—stress has been shown to enhance the immune system, in much the same way that sunlight has positive short-term effects. But those positive effects soon turn sour once stress becomes chronic.) One study compared people caring for a sick relative with a control group who didn't have that responsibility. The caregivers had significantly delayed healing of a skin biopsy by 24 percent in comparison with the control group.[11] Experiments with mice have even discovered a link between chronic stress and a higher risk of developing skin cancer. Scientists at the Johns Hopkins Kimmel Cancer Center found that stressed-out rodents exposed to UV light developed skin cancer in less than half the time it took for nonstressed mice to do so.[12]

When the cortisol level rises during stress, it triggers the sebaceous glands to produce more oil, and the by-product can be acne. Stress also amps up inflammatory reactions, which can make acne worse. A 2002 Stanford University study involving twenty-two students suffering from acne proved that exam stress worsened their conditions. Subjects who had the greatest increases in stress during examination periods also had the greatest exacerbation in acne severity.[13]

To top it off, long-term stress can also age us. In 2004, a study found that the white blood cells of mothers caring for chronically ill children aged more rapidly than those of the control group (mothers with healthy children). The women who perceived themselves to be under high psychological stress (even if they did not have sick children) also had accelerated cellular aging.[14] If all this isn't enough to motivate us to start meditating or doing yoga, I don't know what is. All of these stress responses have even inspired the creation of an entirely new medical field called "psychodermatology" that specializes in using meditation, psychotherapy, and even antidepressants in conjunction with dermatologic medicine. In my office, I'm very quick to offer the business card of an excellent psychotherapist whom I trust. I tell my patients that she can help with stress of all kinds, and I recommend that other medical doctors do the same. I think your doctor should be as concerned about your mental health as your physical well-being; they are linked together inextricably.

External Factors

Smoking

I have to take just one look at somebody to tell that he or she smokes. The fine lines around the lips and the rough, thicker texture and dull color of the skin are glaring signs. I know I'm stating the blatantly obvious when I say smoking is bad for you, but it really does have a disastrous impact on the skin (as if all the other warnings weren't enough). Smoking induces intrinsic changes, such as causing the blood vessels to constrict. That peripheral vasoconstriction of the tiny vessels close to the surface basically starves the cells of oxygen. (That's why many smokers have such sallow, dull complexions.) Since the engine for cellular rebuilding runs on oxygen, those skin cells die and aren't regenerated as quickly as normal. When you have a wound of any kind on your skin, for example, it won't heal as fast as it should. For that reason, I always tell my patients who smoke to stop for two to four weeks after skin surgery. Often they even quit forever!

We all know that smoking is an enormous risk factor for heart and lung diseases as well as many kinds of terminal cancers. But the smoke fumes are carcinogenic externally, too. Because it creates a buildup of toxins around your face and mouth and damages the DNA in skin tissue, smoking is also associated with the development of skin cancer. Recent studies have found that it triples the risk for squamous cell carcinoma. In the eighteenth century there was a huge incidence of scrotum squamous cell carcinoma in chimney sweeps. The toxic char from the chimneys was deadly. In this century, studies have suggested that air pollution—and ozone-depleting atmospheric chemicals—is a significant environmental risk factor for skin cancers too. One 1995 study asserts that the skin is the site of significant absorption of environmental pollutants.[15]

It's obvious that the act of smoking, one's own personal pollution, overuses certain muscles of the face, creating wrinkles around the mouth, frown lines between the eyes, and crow's feet from squinting. The carcinogens in tobacco smoke also kill off collagen, so a smoker's skin becomes wrinkled and less elastic before its time. It's been proven that cigarette smoke degrades collagen and elastin (in a similar, lethal way as ultraviolet rays do) and decreases cell turnover in the skin.[16] What more do you need to hear? If the danger of skin (and other) cancers isn't motivation enough to kick the habit, now we know that smoking makes you look old faster too.

The Sun

The sun has such an extraordinary direct impact on the skin that chapters 5 and 7 are dedicated to the subject. But in a nutshell, imagine the sun's rays as being like a laser gun, disintegrating your collagen and destroying your cells' DNA. It's almost that simple. The sun can be blamed for over one million new cancers each year, affecting approximately one in seventy people. One in every five people will develop skin cancer during his or her lifetime. How does this wonderful-feeling, beautiful sunshine wreak such havoc? The short UVB wavelengths hit the epidermis and cause sunburns, the obvious immediate sign of sun damage. The longer UVA rays penetrate further into the dermis, causing not only a suntan (a sign of trauma) but premature aging (those rays dissolve collagen and elastin) and skin cancers. The Skin Cancer Foundation reports that more than 90 percent of skin cancers are caused by sun exposure. The National Cancer Institute adds that skin cancer is the most common form of cancer in the United States, with more than one million skin cancers diagnosed annually. These alarming findings are just the beginning, I'm afraid, but the good news is that skin cancer is truly one of the most preventable and curable diseases. I will go into the details of how to protect your skin and thwart this potentially lethal disease in chapter 7.

>>> q&a

Q: If the sun is so bad for my skin, why does my complexion always clear up and improve when I'm on vacation and go out in the sun?

A: It does sound contradictory, but I too experienced the same thing on a family vacation. I usually have dry, sensitive skin and had been breaking out around my mouth and chin. Within one day of going to Florida (leaving the cold weather of New York behind), my acne was completely gone. Within a day of coming back, so did my pimples. It's a profound response to sunlight and to a very different environment (warm, sunny, and humid versus the cold, dry Manhattan winter).

The fact is that sun *does* cause injury to your skin *and* can effect a positive anti-inflammatory response too. Like most things in the medicinal world, a little bit of sun can be good, but too much is very bad. Initially ultraviolet wavelengths penetrate the epidermis and interact with the Langerhans cells (those air traffic controllers directing the immune system) to shut them off temporarily. This stops the immune system from working at its best. Now, some skin diseases, such as psoriasis, acne, and eczema, happen because your inflammatory system is in overdrive. So the UV light helps quell the immune system's overreaction temporarily so the skin can normalize again. (In fact, UV light treatment in a doctor's office is a standard medical prescription for psoriasis.) But the sun soon becomes toxic once the wavelengths begin tanning or burning the skin (on fair skin types this can happen right away), and those rays can actually start killing the Langerhans cells and damaging the immune system. How long it takes to become dangerous depends on your skin type (whether it's fair or darker).

A 2004 study published in the *Journal of the American Academy of Dermatology* found that soaking up UV rays is actually addicting. (So maybe the term "tanorexic" isn't so off the mark.) It's believed that exposure to ultraviolet light leads to a release of endorphins, powerful mood-enhancing chemicals that make a person feel relaxed. In a 2006 study published in the same journal, frequent tanners who were given naltrexone, a drug that blocks the opiate-like endorphins produced in the skin by UV radiation, suffered from physical withdrawal symptoms similar to withdrawal from drugs, cigarettes, or alcohol. Addiction is dangerous, any way you cut it, and a tanning addiction can be as self-destructive and potentially life-threatening as any other habit.

Environment

Because it's our Gore-tex, skin is the first shield to a lot of external influences. It's directly affected by the weather that's around it. A humid atmosphere, for example, brings moisture in the air to the surface of the skin. Often, severely dry skin is directly caused by the climate in which you live. Wind, cold, and dry air steal moisture from the epidermis, making it dangerously dry. At a high altitude the air is drier and you lose most of the water from your skin, which in turn makes the cells shrink (think of a dry sponge) and causes gaps or tiny cracks. The medical term for parched skin like this is actually quite poetic: "eczema craquelé," or "marred with cracks."

>>> q&a

Q: I live in a place that's hot and humid in the summer and cold and dry in the winter. What's the best way to deal with the changing seasons for my skin?

A: Using common sense and adjusting your skin care products are the keys. With every season, reclassify your skin "type" and reevaluate your regimen based on that. Your skin will let you know what it needs: Is it feeling oily, dry, or irritated? Is it breaking out much more? In a warm, humid climate you may want to use an oil-free sunscreen as your daily moisturizer and apply a lightweight moisturizer at night before bed. If you have oily skin, you may be able to skip moisturizer at night altogether. Simply put, unless your skin is extremely dry, it's getting moisture from the air and not losing as much water either. You're not producing more oil (although it sure feels like it); you're just not losing the moisture that you already have in your epidermis. You can use an astringent toner (containing witch hazel or alcohol) to clean especially oily areas of your face. Humidity is actually hydrating and very healthy for your skin (although it doesn't always feel like it on a hot day when you're sweating up a storm). And remember that sweating is the body's biofeedback mechanism to cool you off.

It's dry air that causes trouble. Cold, dry air does a number on your skin as the humidity drops. Use a creamy lotion cleanser and a richer moisturizer containing humectants (such as hyaluronic acid or glycerin) to attract whatever moisture is in the atmosphere and occlusive emollients like squalene to seal it in. Using a humidifier in your home is a great antidote in an arid atmosphere too. (Radiator heat is an unbeatable dehydrating force on your skin.) Also, cut bathing time down to the bare minimum and make sure the water is warm, not hot. As wonderful as a long hot bath or shower feels on a cold day, it's dehydrating in the extreme. Don't forget to follow it up by moisturizing with a rich body lotion or cream.

>>> skin lie: Spraying water on your face adds moisture to your skin in the dry atmosphere of an airplane.

>>> skin truth: No way. It's true that the low-humidity, dry-air environment inside a pressurized plane cabin is totally moisture-sapping. (There's usually 10 percent less moisture on a plane than inside your house.) Your skin and lips, even your eyes, become very dry almost immediately. But misting water on your face intermittently throughout a long flight will actually make matters worse because your skin will be even dryer once the water evaporates. If you like to use a facial mist, make sure it contains something more than H_2O—a humectant ingredient such as glycerin or aloe vera, which will lock on the moisture you just spritzed and will keep your skin hydrated. Try not to drink alcohol or eat salty foods, which dehydrate you even more, and make sure to drink enough water (more for your internal systems than for your skin).

It's also essential to apply a rich moisturizer (a facial mist alone won't be enough for arid conditions like these), and if you are traveling in daylight hours, make sure the product has a sunblock ingredient in it. The UV rays are far more intense at higher altitudes (the thinner, higher air doesn't screen out as much harmful radiation), so you have to contend with the double whammy of dehydration and sun damage. Sunblock inside an airplane? Yes.

Your Own Skin Care Products

You can file this one under "can't win for losing," but the products you put on your skin to make it more beautiful may actually be causing your problems. On any given day, the average woman uses at least twenty-five different products on her skin, containing hundreds of chemicals (both synthetic and natural). They obviously influence how oily or dry your skin feels. They can also cause irritation or even allergic reactions and may clog your pores and cause acne. *And* it's possible that they may interact with one another and become more harmful. Something as simple as what you use to wash your face, or the way you wash it, can create a host of complexion troubles. Washing too much (especially with a cleanser containing drying detergents, alcohol-based gel formulations, or salicylic acid) can dry out your skin. By the same token, oil-based cleansers or creams (and oil-based makeup) can cause breakouts.

Some people are genetically inclined toward sensitive skin, but we all have the potential to acquire it. Overdoing products that break down the stratum corneum cause irritant contact dermatitis and will trigger an immune response as part of the body's healing mechanism. For instance, mixing and matching different skin care products can cause serious inflammation. Stacking up a retinoid plus a glycolic acid cleanser and an alpha-hydroxy acid (AHA) moisturizer increases their strength threefold. All of those things are meant to dissolve something on the top part of your skin, so basically you are giving yourself a chemical peel every night. Even if you use over-the-counter-strength lotions and cleansers, piling on several of them could leave you with a rash rather than the glowing complexion you're trying to acquire. I frequently see patients who have dry, red, flaking skin around their nose and mouth or near their eyes, and a lot of the time it's from using too many hard-core ingredients. These are the smart but confused patients who inspired me to write this book. The main objective of your daily regimen is to maintain the protective surface of your skin. If you use too many acids and harsh products, you erode that layer and expose yourself to infections and strip the stratum corneum of moisture. Again, you have to read your skin, be careful, and be sensible about what you apply on top of it. Stop. Simplify. Learn. Start a smarter system.

>>> skin lie: Washing your face excessively can make it oilier because sebaceous glands go into overdrive trying to moisturize the skin.

>>> skin truth: There are definitely amazing biofeedback mechanisms going on in your skin all the time. Those tireless inflammatory cells go into action to repair the stratum corneum when it is wounded by a sunburn, a scrape, or excessive dryness caused by too much washing, which strips the skin of natural oils. But I don't think those internal systems are so specific that they would stimulate oil production on parched skin, and no research makes this claim. (Otherwise there would be no dry skin problems to contend with, right?) Dry skin may instigate pimple production, however, as an inflammatory stress reaction. And drying out the skin may clog pores with dead keratinocytes (which helps to create an acne situation), but it doesn't activate the sebaceous glands.

4

Your Seriously Simple Skin Care Plan

Let's start with the basics. There are only three products you *need* to use on your skin every day: a gentle cleanser, a moisturizer, and a sunscreen. And depending on how your skin is behaving, that number could be cut down to just one: sunscreen. Your regimen does not have to take more than a few minutes or cost more than a few dollars. Most of the time, the best thing you can do for your complexion is the least amount necessary. There are many smart reasons to use very little on your skin, and most of the time your amazing body can take care of itself. A minimalist approach exposes your skin to fewer chemicals (which is a safe thing), and by reducing the steps in your daily regimen, the more compliant and successful you'll be at maintaining it. It's a little like going on an intense diet; you'll never keep up that kind of complex discipline for long.

You also have to be willing to change your routine as necessary. Your medicine chest should be armed with a small, but mighty, arsenal of products (the three basics and two or three extras) that you can pull out in an emergency, such as an acne flare-up or a rash. First, do a quick analysis of your skin every day: Is my T-zone breaking out? Does my skin feel particularly oily or dry? Is it irritated? Then be practical. If your face is red and irritated (perhaps it's because you've been using a particular product or the environment is especially dry or cold), you should moisturize it with something mild. The last thing you want to do is scrub irritated skin or apply any kind of acid on top of it (whether citric, AHA, or salicylic). Be sensible, and err on the side of doing less—or nothing at all—because, given a few days, your skin may heal itself.

A regimen is the solution to what your skin requires on any given day. The goal of this low-maintenance routine is simple: to maintain the stratum corneum. This means keeping it clean, hydrated, and protected. Despite all the advertisements and beauty articles to the contrary, skin truly needs the barest minimum: a gentle cleanser (and in a pinch warm water alone will do just fine), a moisturizer (and if you have oily skin, skip it entirely), and, most important of all, sunscreen or sunblock. Everyone at every age needs to use sun protection every single day (yes, on cloudy days too). It's by far the most effective and significant thing you can do to protect your skin and prevent sun damage, skin cancer, and premature aging.

If you use only one product, make it a sunblock and use it every day.

So where should you begin? Even choosing three everyday basics can be overwhelming. In this chapter I'll explain which formulations (lotions, creams, gels, balms, and more) will work best for your skin, and I'll clear up the mystery of confusing cosmetic ingredients so you can understand what you're purchasing and putting on your skin. But first you need to know what kind of skin you tend to have.

Skin Detox

Many times patients come to see me with red, flaky, irritated skin on their face or neck. Sometimes this is due to just one product that is obviously creating an allergic reaction. In this case, we do a patch test to discover which ingredients may be the cause. Or they may be stripping their skin (in an effort to fight one or two pimples or to "correct" an oily T-zone) by washing too much or overusing drying ingredients such as alcohol or salicylic acid. In that case, the skin isn't given a chance to generate the oil necessary to protect itself, and the epidermal barrier may be compromised. Most often irritation happens when a person uses too many serums, potions, and lotions (possibly layering on a glycolic, citric, or salicylic acid product after using an AHA cleanser or on top of an antioxidant serum or under some other kind of something-or-other). Piling all those chemicals on the skin (and yes, even in a pretty package, even all natural, and with a whipped-cream consistency, these are chemicals) can set you up for serious irritation. Using too much of a good thing isn't going to make the skin look better.

In response to skin irritation (whether from an allergic reaction or product overkill) or when someone simply has no idea what kind of basics his or her skin may need, I have the same radical plan of action: stop everything at once. Your skin needs to get back to its natural balance or imbalance with no intervention from topical chemicals. Only then can any skin evaluation be accurate. You should still use a sunscreen and (only if you have to) a gentle cleanser and a moisturizer containing no active ingredients such as retinoids, acids, or antioxidants. Detox from as much as possible, including makeup if you can handle it (eye makeup and mascara are okay), so that you can see what your skin issues really are, without taking it in one direction or another with products. How long do you have to practice this cosmetic abstinence? One month. That's right, one month. It takes about twenty-eight days for your skin to go through a complete growth cycle (the basal cells maturing all the way up to the surface and then dying and sloughing off). I know it seems harsh and unnecessary, but I promise you, so are most of the things you've been using on your face. Consider it tough love.

You might slowly add one product back into your routine per week. This way, if your skin reacts, it will be easier to identify the cause of this irritation. Now you can figure out exactly what kind of essentials your skin should have.

Should you pick a milky cleanser or a gel? Do you need a very emollient moisturizer or none at all? Should you look for a sunblock with physical blockers rather than a chemical sunscreen? Now that you can read your skin clearly, I can help you with the answers.

The Delivery System

It's not just the active ingredients (the ones that directly do something for your skin, such as sunblocks, acids, antioxidants, and retinoids) that matter when it comes to a cosmetic. The "delivery system" or "vehicle" in which they are applied to your skin is equally important because it makes up the majority of the product as a whole. Most of the ingredients in any product are inactive. Their secondary function is to benefit the skin directly. These substances work together to create a base that carries the active ingredients (a moisturizer, detergent, or sunscreen), and, as a by-product, they can also benefit the skin. Some of these (especially certain preservatives) may be potentially irritating. I'll discuss those in more detail in the next few pages. These inactive ingredients make a cream glide on smoothly or help a cleanser lather up. They are the preservatives that prevent the product from decomposing and make it resistant to bacteria, or the buffers that control its acidity and pH balance. There are thickening agents, and there are emulsifiers that allow oily and water-based materials to mix so ingredients don't separate. Some ingredients create the color of a product, and some make it smell nice. Each has an important function, and many have multiple jobs, as you'll see in the ingredients list later in this chapter. So "inactive" is something of a misnomer; these are very functional ingredients indeed.

Before we tackle specific ingredients and more complex label decoding, let's stick with the essential consistency of a product or its vehicle. That's an easy guide to choosing a product compatible with your skin (remember, you may need to switch the formulation if your skin changes seasonally or for any other reason). For example, if you tend to have a dry complexion most of the time, a creamy cleanser and an emollient-based moisturizer will be friendlier to your skin than an alcohol-based gel cleanser and a light water-based lotion. But if your complexion gets oilier during the humid months of summer, you might want to give the water-based moisturizer a try and put the richer cream away for the season.

When you are picking a product, think about your lifestyle. Do you spend a lot of time outdoors? (You'll need a stronger sunblock if you do.) Do you live in a humid climate? (You should try water-based or gel formulations and perhaps skip moisturizer altogether.) Think about what you're already doing regimen-wise. Which products are you always reaching for? An astringent to degrease your skin or a moisturizer because your face feels taut most of the time?

Generally, the lighter a product's formulation (a liquid, lotion, gel, or foam), the better it will be for oily or acne-prone skin. Usually these vehicles are water- or alcohol-based. They tend to evaporate from the skin and provide a little less hydration and staying power. Creams, balms and thicker lotions are usually oil or wax-based. These are the best bets for dry skin because they occlude it, creating another barrier over the skin's surface with ingredients such as mineral oil, shea butter, lanolin, or petrolatum. It's a good idea to double-check the ingredients in any product to make sure they're compatible with your skin. For example, a cleanser containing a detergent such as sodium laureth sulfate will probably irritate dry skin, but oily skin may need this stronger surfactant, the "surface-acting agent" that breaks down oil and washes it away.

The Bare Essentials

Your Facial Cleanser

I admit it, usually I don't use cleanser at all. My skin is dry and sensitive, so it doesn't produce a lot of oil, and I don't wear much makeup. So for me, warm water and a washcloth work just fine. The point of a cleanser is to clean off the oil, debris, and makeup that accrue during a normal day, and to do that you don't need anything harsh or too powerful. All soaps or detergents work by a process called "micellation," which breaks down big substances (such as oil or dirt) into smaller ones using a chemical reaction, so they can rinse off the skin easily. A fatty-acid ingredient attaches to the oils on the skin and dissolves them, while an alkaline element makes it possible to rinse it all off the skin. Micellation works best using warm water, about the same temperature as your body, simply because it's more compatible with the cleanser and with your skin.

By the way, most of us aren't technically using soap. Traditionally, soap is made from either vegetable oil or animal fat and lye (otherwise known as sodium hydroxide, a water-soluble alkali that emulsifies in water). Today, most cleansers (including products that are loosely defined as "soap") use synthetic detergents, which are cheaper and easier to manufacture and tend to be gentler because they are less alkaline. The normal pH of the skin is between 4.5 and 6.5, and an alkaline substance raises that level, increasing the potential for dryness and irritation. They both work in the same way, which is why many cleansers leave the skin feeling dry, since their job is to literally wash away oils from the surface.

Surfactants

Every cleanser contains a surfactant, which emulsifies and washes debris and oil from the skin. This may seem obvious, but their names are not. I'm sure most of us wouldn't know the difference between sodium lauryl sulfate and sodium cocyl isethionate (or how to pronounce them!), but there is actually a big distinction (the first is a stronger detergent and the second is mild). We've always heard that the more a cleanser foams, the more drying it will be, and that's partially true, primarily because it likely contains a larger quantity of detergent. Here's a quick list of the most common cleansing agents, but it's not just the surfactant that makes a cleanser extra-drying, it's also the other active and inactive ingredients in the vehicle. And often there may be more than one kind of surfactant in a single cleanser. So keep in mind that a cleanser containing a gentle cleansing agent may still dry out your skin if it also includes salicylic acid or alcohol.

Cleansing Ingredients

>>> SOAP COMPOUNDS
(BETTER FOR OILY SKIN AND REMOVING HEAVY MAKEUP)

Sodium tallowate

Sodium cocoate

Sodium palm kernelate

Sodium palmate or palmitate

>>> HARSHER SYNTHETIC SURFACTANTS
(BETTER FOR OILY SKIN AND REMOVING HEAVY MAKEUP)

Sodium lauryl sulfate

Sodium dodecylbenzene sulfonate

>>> MILD SYNTHETIC SURFACTANTS
(BETTER FOR NORMAL, DRY, OR SENSITIVE SKIN)

Sodium laureth sulfate

Sodium cocyl isethionate

Cocomidopropyl betaine

Disodium cocamphodiacetate

Ammonium lauryl sulfate

Sodium lauroyl isenthionate or sarcosinate

Lauric acid diethenolamine (lauramide DEA)

Caprylic acid (derived from coconuts; often used in natural and organic products)

Sodium cocoyl glutamate (derived from coconuts; often used in natural and organic products)

Polysorbate 85 or polysorbate 60 (a gentle, moisturizing surfactant created from the plant-derived emollient sorbitol)

Soap: A Mini-glossary

With so many variations on a very simple idea—how to clean your skin—it's hard to keep things straight. What is a "nonsoap cleanser"? What's the difference between "antibacterial" and "glycerin" soap? Are "natural" cleansers really so different from the synthetic brands? Here are the simple facts about soaps.

Soap. Soap is a salt of a fatty acid, made from vegetable oils or butters (such as palm or coconut) or animal fat ingredients (such as lard) and an alkali salt (lye or sodium hydroxide). Often you will see the term "sodium cocoate" on a soap, which is the mix of sodium hydroxide and coconut oil. "Sodium tallowate" is the combination of sodium hydroxide and animal fat. True soaps can be drying and irritating to skin.

Synthetic detergents. Often referred to as "syndet bars" or "soap-free" soaps, these use synthetic—and usually milder—surfactants such as sodium cocyl isethionate (which is derived from coconuts) or sodium palmitate. Since they utilize less alkaline salts in their surfactants, these have a much lower pH, which makes them less irritating. Dove, the very first syndet bar introduced in 1955, is made primarily from sodium lauroyl isethionate but contains sodium tallowate and palmitate too. Many liquid facial cleansers use only synthetic surfactants (such as sodium laureth sulfate, the prime detergent in Clinique Liquid Facial Soap).

Combination bars. These combine real soap with synthetic detergents (as you might expect, they are less irritating than pure soap but not as mild as a synthetic detergent). They lather up better and have a stronger cleansing action than milder syndet bars. Gentle cleansers, such as Cetaphil and the aforementioned Dove, are examples of combination bars. Cetaphil contains sodium tallowate, sodium cocoate, and sodium cocyl isethionate (a mild synthetic surfactant), among other detergents.

Glycerin soap. This is a transparent soap with added glycerin (a vegetable oil moisturizing agent). Products such as Neutrogena's Transparent Facial Bar, for instance, may be milder and more moisturizing due to the glycerin, but they still contain soap ingredients such as sodium cocoate and tallowate.

Antibacterial soap. This is any synthetic detergent or soap with added antibacterial ingredients, such as triclosan, tetrasodium EDTA, triclocarbon, or plain alcohol. Dial Antibacterial Hand Soap, for example, is a liquid cleanser that contains synthetic surfactants—sodium laureth sulfate and ammonium lauryl sulfate—and 0.15% of the antibacterial ingredient triclosan to kill germs and bacteria. These can irritate the skin, and an FDA advisory panel says that they are no more effective in preventing illness than plain old soap and water.

Deodorant soap. This usually contains soap plus antibacterial ingredients such as tetrasodium EDTA. Because the goal is to deodorize, they may add synthetic fragrance and usually a combination of both soap and synthetic detergents. Lever 2000 Deodorant Soap is made from sodium tallowate, sodium cocoate, and sodium palm kernelate and adds tetrasodium EDTA and a fragrance. (Natural deodorant soap options include sage and rosemary extracts or lemongrass oil to control odor.)

Natural soap. This contains mild, sulfate-free surfactants (such as sodium cocoyl glutamate, caprylic acid or sodium lauroyl, from coconuts and amino acids, respectively), derived from the same natural sources as regular soap and synthetic detergents. Tom's of Maine Natural (Unscented) Moisturizing Body Bar uses soap from coconut and palm oils, and—like most natural soaps—includes no synthetic detergents, animal fats, artificial preservatives, or perfumes. The processing of these ingredients is presumably (but not necessarily) more environmentally sound and less chemical-based. (See "Natural and Organic Skin Care: The Butterfly Effect" on page 103 for more information.)

Besides the *type* of cleanser you use, the *amount* of washing you do is important. Unless you have very oily skin, there's no need to wash your face more than once a day, especially if you have dry skin. Cleanse at the end of the day to remove grime, sweat, makeup, and oil. It's unlikely that your skin will get too greasy or dirty overnight, so rinsing it with water in the morning (rather than rewashing) is all that's necessary. And it won't strip your skin of its healthy supply of natural oils that protect the skin's epidermal barrier. Splashing *cold* water on your face in the morning is especially refreshing. It causes vasoconstriction of the vessels and brightens your complexion, and it makes your pores look tighter. (It's no wonder that movie stars like Joan Crawford used this ice water trick every morning.)

With all the options available—lathering cleansers, bar soaps, non-foaming washes, and even cleansing oils—here are basic guidelines for choosing the best kind of cleanser to suit the skin you tend to have.

THE RIGHT TYPES OF FACIAL CLEANSERS TO USE

IF YOUR SKIN TENDS TO BE DRY

Remember that, for you, using warm water and a washcloth can be enough to clean your face. Dry skin lacks excess oil on the stratum corneum, so the worst thing you can do is use a strong detergent or soap. You want less soap and more moisturizer. Try using a cleanser with an extra-gentle surfactant such as polysorbate 85 or 60, coc-amidropropyl betaine, or caprylic acid, and make sure it has added humectants and emollients. Humectants, such as glycerin and hy-aluronic acid, attract water and help the skin retain it. Occlusive emol-lients, such as squalene and coconut oil, are lubricating, waxy thick ingredients that hold moisture on the skin. Look for formulations such as creamy lotion or cleansing milk. You're also a great candidate for a cold cream cleanser, a cleansing oil, or a balm; they basically act on the same gentle cleansing principle. (Take a look at the Q&A on page 66 for more information.)

IF YOUR SKIN TENDS TO BE OILY OR ACNE-PRONE

When your skin is oily, you want to use micellation to dissolve and wash away the overload of oil. You can use soap or a slightly more powerful synthetic detergent such as sodium lauryl sulfate or even sodium laureth sulfate, and consider a cleanser that has 2 percent sali-cylic acid as a component. This will dissolve the dead keratin cells plugging the pores and help prevent acne. A facial wash that also con-tains benzoyl peroxide, an antibacterial agent, will prevent bacteria from overpopulating in the pores (another facet of acne production). Usually over-the-counter cleansers contain no more than 2.5 percent benzoyl peroxide. Both of these ingredients are extremely drying, and most "acne washes" should be used only if you truly have oily skin. If you have one or two zits and an oily T-zone, this kind of cleanser will leave your skin totally parched. (If an oily T-zone is your issue, read the Q&A on page 67.) Stick with water or alcohol-based gels, foaming liquids, or lotions. FYI, cleansers for oily skin usually have terms such as "purifying" or "clarifying" on the label. Stay far away from emollients such as squalene and mineral oil. For you, using them is basically putting oil on top of oil. If you have acne-prone skin, the more diligent you are about daily maintenance and cleansing, the less acne you will have. But do not obsess about constantly stripping oil from your skin; oil is still healthy.

IF YOUR SKIN TENDS TO BE SENSITIVE

People with sensitive skin run the gamut from those with a fair-skinned, delicate complexion, to someone with rosacea or with dark skin that is prone to hyperpigmentation. Essentially, when dealing with skin that gets red and irritated easily, burns quickly in the sun, or is susceptible to dark spots, you must use care and caution. Minimize your use of products to the point of applying nearly nothing to your skin. A less-of-everything routine doesn't tamper with the barrier function of the stratum corneum. As with dry skin, don't wash it more than once per day, and use gentle formulations (cleansing lotions or milks) with the mildest surfactants. Gels and oil-free washes usually clean away too much oil, but a creamier cleanser will replenish the healthy lipids on the surface. (Most people with sensitive skin tend to have rosacea or dryness too.) Occlusive emollients in a cleanser or moisturizer help protect sensitive skin by creating a stronger surface barrier. It's also important to look for anti-inflammatory ingredients, such as soy, allantoin, aloe vera, or chamomile. These will soothe the skin and calm redness. I tend to have sensitive skin, so I use a face wash (Terralina Gentle Cleanser) that contains chamomile and oat extract, the natural emollient olive oil and humectants (such as glycerin).

I advise my patients with even slightly sensitive skin to always patch test a new product before using it on the face. (This goes for any new cleanser, sunscreen, moisturizer, makeup, scrub, anything at all.) Remember they could interact with each other and irritate your skin. Try it out on your inner wrist or forearm, since the skin there is thin and more similar to facial skin. And be patient: you need to test a product for four days in a row. This way, if the product doesn't trigger a reaction immediately, you'll be able to see if repeated applications cause irritation. It is not unusual to have a delayed allergic reaction that may not show up for weeks. Also, realize that your cheeks have a higher concentration of blood vessels, so you might react differently there no matter how much pretesting you do. The creases around the nose and eyes are particularly sensitive because products accumulate there in higher concentrations.

>>> q&a

Q: Won't an oil cleanser make my skin break out? How do they work?

A: It very well could make you break out if you have oily skin or acne on a regular basis. In that case, you're better off with a water-based, oil-free facial wash. But someone with sensitive or dry skin will do very well with this formulation because it leaves a little healthy oil on the skin after washing away makeup or grime. Think of makeup, dirt, sweat, and sebum on your face at the end of the day as dried paint (beautifully applied and natural-looking dried paint, of course). To make it easier to clean off that dried-up debris, you need something to wet it again. Cleansing oil is oil-soluble, meaning it's compatible with the other oils and makeup ingredients on your face. It's able to bind with that residue, loosen it, and make it easier to lift off the face. It's similar to using a cold cream or an oily makeup remover. Some oil-based cleansers also contain a super-gentle surfactant, such as polysorbate 80, to help the emulsification process along. Another big positive with cleansing oil is that you tend to massage it into your skin for much longer than you would a foaming cleanser. This stimulates circulation and dilates the vessels on top of the dermis. Massaging the face delivers oxygen and nourishment to the skin (through the dilated blood vessels). And it feels good too.

Q: I have a very oily T-zone, so I often break out in the middle of my face, especially on my nose and chin. But the skin on my cheeks is normal to dry. Do I need different products for oily skin and dry skin?

A: You are actually quite lucky if you have this kind of complexion, because it's resilient. You can use almost anything you want on it. I consider combination skin like yours to be the closest thing to a "normal" skin type. Because your skin is neither too oily, too dry, nor too sensitive, feel free to use whatever formulations or ingredients you prefer. You can buy something because it smells good or the packaging appeals to you without worrying about the effect it might have because your skin recovers so easily. It's probably a good idea in general to choose products that say "noncomedogenic" on the label, because they don't tend to clog pores with emollients such as mineral oil (an ingredient you don't need on oily areas). I'm not a fan of toners in general and don't think they're usually necessary, but in your case an astringent toner is a fine way to degrease the T-zone without drying the entire face. You want to look for a toner geared to oily or acne-prone skin, with ingredients like alcohol, witch hazel extract, lactic acid, or salicylic acid. All these strip the skin of oil and help keep pores clean of dead skin cells, but they're also extremely drying. Use this kind of toner only on the oily areas of your face.

Q: If I wash my face with facial wash containing glycolic acid or benzoyl peroxide, will it do anything at all, since the acid is so diluted with water while I'm washing and rinses right off?

A: A cleanser containing active ingredients such as AHA acids, salicylic acid, or benzoyl peroxide will definitely have an effect. Usually a cleanser containing any of these ingredients uses a stronger surfactant, so it will leave the skin very dry. Acids work immediately, so if you use a cleanser with 2 percent salicylic acid, that active ingredient does its job (dissolving dead cells on the surface of skin) the minute it interacts with the skin. It doesn't need to sit on your face for long. Even though you wash it off, a residual of an active ingredient such as benzoyl peroxide will linger on the skin and remain active and effective.

>>> skin lie: Washcloths breed bacteria and can therefore cause skin conditions such as acne or folliculitis.

>>> skin truth: I'm a huge believer in the washcloth. I think a nubby washcloth is one of your best skin care tools. It's a good way to slough off dead skin cells while you wash your face and much less abrasive and irritating than a facial scrub or a chemical exfoliant for someone with a tendency toward dry or sensitive skin. A clean washcloth should not harbor bacteria, in the same way that your toothbrush, if it's stored properly and allowed to dry out, won't become a breeding ground either. Granted, if you store a wet cloth in a damp place, you're going to have problems, but squeezing out the extra moisture and then hanging it to dry on your towel rack should be safe. Most bacteria can't live in a dry environment, so if you let your cloth air out in between uses, it will be absolutely fine for a few days. Rinse it with soap before you hang it to dry. If it smells mildewy after a few wet-to-dry uses, it's time to change it. A natural sponge or a loofah can also be an effective exfoliating tool. (Since these tend to be a little large, you can cut them into smaller, flatter pieces, making it easier for them to dry out completely in between uses.) If you're still not convinced, try a disposable cleansing cloth product, one with the cleanser integrated into the fibers. The cloth will foam up once it's dampened and you can start washing, then toss the cloth. Since you use a clean cloth every time, there's no chance for residue or bacteria to build up, not to mention that they're convenient for traveling since they aren't actually considered a liquid. But the environmentalist in me thinks these are wasteful and not the best choice.

Your Facial Moisturizer

Think of the skin's surface like the paint job on a car. If the paint is cracked, the metal underneath is left unprotected from the elements and quickly oxidizes and rusts. The same concept goes for your stratum corneum—once it's dry, brittle, or cracked, you've lost your shield and the skin is vulnerable to exposure from the outside and water evaporates from the dermis. You can get fissures on the skin, and infections can easily occur. When the barrier function is compromised for any reason (trauma, wind, dry air, too many chemicals on your skin), bacteria enters the dermis through the cracks on the surface. The stratum corneum contains approximately 30 percent water and lipids. Its water content is essential, even though it's made up of dead cells. If that Gore-tex dries out completely, it can't protect the layers of skin underneath. Similar to the shiny, beautiful coating on a car's exterior, putting on moisturizer not only makes the surface look pretty, it seals and protects what is beneath it.

During the day, even the darkest, dreariest one, your facial moisturizer must contain a sunscreen. End of story. No arguments. At night, after cleansing your skin, there's obviously no reason to use sun protection, but there's a great need to replenish the lipids that just went down the drain when you washed your face. It's the same rationale as the application of a body lotion after a shower: replacing the natural oils that were rinsed off. Unfortunately, I often see patients who rarely if ever apply a moisturizer anywhere, and the result is itchy, red, flaky skin that leaves them vulnerable to infections. For most of us, except those with very oily skin, moisturizer shouldn't be thought of as an indulgence. It is crucial to keeping your skin's defenses up.

Moisturizers use two types of hydrating ingredients: humectants, which attract water molecules to the skin, and emollients, which seal that moisture on top by forming an occlusive protective barrier. There are usually plenty of both in a single moisturizer, and, as you'll see in the following ingredients list, many humectant and emollient substances are multitaskers, used to make the vehicle more effective. Their primary function may be to make the lotion creamier or better able to glide onto the skin, but they also have a secondary hydrating benefit. Here is a list of the most common humectants and emollients found in almost any moisturizer on the market, from the priciest cream to a basic drugstore lotion.

Moisturizer Ingredients

>>> HUMECTANTS (ATTRACT WATER)

Glycerin

Hyaluronic acid

Propylene glycol

Butylene glycol

Sodium PCA

Sorbitol

Allantoin

>>> OCCLUSIVE EMOLLIENTS (CREATE A PROTECTIVE BARRIER)

Shea butter

Mineral oil

Lanolin

Petrolatum

Paraffin

Beeswax

Squalene

Coconut, jojoba, and sesame oils

Cetyl alcohol

As long as your moisturizer contains some of these, your skin will be healthy and protected. Do you need a heavier, thicker formulation at night? No. Just use a consistency similar to that of your daytime moisturizer, but without the sunscreen. Unless your skin is dry, it doesn't have to be richer to be more effective. Use these guidelines to help select the right ingredients and formulations of moisturizer for how your skin usually acts.

THE RIGHT TYPES OF FACIAL MOISTURIZERS TO USE

IF YOUR SKIN TENDS TO BE DRY

The natural oils and lipids that should be in the epidermis are in short supply, so dry skin is desperate for humectants and emollients. It will drink up a rich, heavy-duty moisturizer, such as a lotion or cream that's oil-based (a water-based product evaporates quickly and won't provide enough long-lasting moisture). Look for one that has waxy occlusive emollients such as shea butter, squalene, even lanolin or mineral oil. In your case, you may want to use a heavier moisturizer at bedtime (since you don't need to worry about wearing it under makeup and making your skin appear too greasy). Go for it, slather on as much moisture as you need from your forehead down to your collarbone. (No matter how your skin behaves, we all need to remember to treat our neck like our face. That means cleansing, moisturizing, and, most vital of all, protecting it from the sun with sunscreen daily.)

IF YOUR SKIN TENDS TO BE OILY OR ACNE-PRONE

It's important to read your skin accurately, and if it already feels more than moisturized after washing, then skip this step. Why hydrate an already oily surface? There's no point. But if you feel slightly tight (especially if your cleanser contains salicylic acid or a drying detergent), use a water-based, lightweight lotion or gel formulation that contains more humectant ingredients (such as hyaluronic acid or glycerin) than waxy or oily emollients. It's important for you to look for the word "noncomedogenic" on the label. A comedone is a blackhead or whitehead plugging up a pore, and you certainly don't want anything that can contribute to those (namely, occlusive ingredients such as mineral oil, lanolin, or petrolatum). Don't forget sunscreen; at least wear a powder containing a titanium dioxide or zinc oxide sunblock; or try a face wash containing sunscreen ingredients. (See "Sunscreen Formulations" on page 84 for more information about sunscreen facial washes.)

IF YOUR SKIN TENDS TO BE SENSITIVE

Again, it's wise to patch test any new product first, and you must really baby your skin. I mean that literally in that you should choose products almost mild enough to use on a baby's skin. "Fragrance-free" and "hypoallergenic" are two buzzwords to look for on a product's label. It will probably contain fewer irritants, chemicals, and preservatives that can potentially affect your skin in a negative way. The fewer ingredients in any facial product, the gentler and safer it will be for sensitive skin (or for any complexion, for that matter). Avoid extremes; stay away from very heavy emollient creams as well as drying gel formulas, which may contain alcohol. Try a water-based lotion or cream instead. One thing you definitely do want added to your moisturizer is an anti-inflammatory ingredient such as soy, aloe vera, cucumber, calendula, oatmeal, or allantoin. These ingredients may soothe irritated or red skin. Make sure your daily sunscreen, cleanser, and moisturizer do not contain perfumes or acids and have as few chemicals as possible. Use a daily moisturizer with the sunblock titanium dioxide or zinc oxide, which are less irritating than chemical suncreen ingredients.

>>> q&a

Q: Are drugstore products just as good as the pricier brands?

A: Marketing and perception are very powerful forces. A fascinating Duke University study published in 2008 in *The Journal of the Ameri-*

can Medical Association found that people believed that a more expensive placebo pill actually worked better just because it cost more.[1] Go figure. Spending more money somehow convinces many people that something (in this case a drug) works better. If that belief combined with the enjoyment of applying an expensive, more luxurious lotion or sunscreen makes you more inclined to use it with consistency, the placebo effect works wonders.

Logically, however, consider that your three fundamental products all include similar common ingredients (perhaps in slightly varying concentrations). It just doesn't make rational sense to spend more money on them. Cleansers, sunscreens, and basic moisturizers contain about the same kinds of surfactants, humectants, and moisturizing emollients. These products all coat the top of the skin and affect it superficially. And many of the big cosmetics manufacturers (the names you see all over the drugstore aisles) are the same ones that make the prestige beauty lines. All the scientific bells and whistles that increase the cost of a product—tiny nanoparticles that might be able to penetrate further than the surface, a truly stabilized form of an antioxidant such as vitamin C or green tea, or retinoids that would actually break through to the dermis—don't matter so much (from a medical standpoint) for a cleanser, sunscreen, or simple moisturizer. In the upcoming section on cosmeceuticals, I'll discuss certain ingredients that cost more (such as retinoids, stable antioxidants, and plant extracts) and why they may or may not be worth the extra money. But the fact is that the most effective antiaging product on the market is a good sunblock, and that doesn't have to be expensive at all. Honestly, the best, strongest sun protection products can be purchased at the drugstore. The bottom line: it's all a matter of personal preference. If you want to splurge on basics, go ahead, but it's simply not necessary.

Q: Can I mix and match different brands of cleansers and moisturizers?

A: Of course! It's okay as long as you read the fine print. It's far too easy to go overboard with strong ingredients if you're not careful. I see many patients who go for overkill, using too much of a good (or harsh) thing without being aware of it. For example, you may be using a cleanser that contains a salicylic acid, then applying a lotion with some kind of alpha-hydroxy acid (AHA), and not even know it. This kind of overlap and excess can unintentionally cause serious irritation. You must look at the ingredients carefully and then evaluate whether the new product is compatible with your existing regimen or giving you double doses of an active ingredient. (This is important to consider when you receive a free sample at a department store too. Find out what's actually in it before you put it on your face.) For this reason, I think using a skin care system is a rational way to go. A line of products that is made to work together harmoniously is simple to use and will prevent the possibility of exceeding the limit on harsh substances. For someone with sensitivity, this is especially important, because you don't want to keep introducing new ingredients and chemicals to your skin.

Additionally, switching often doesn't give a product with active ingredients a chance to work. Many cosmeceutical ingredients (such as Retin-A or retinols) can take six weeks to take effect. Just because you don't see a noticeable effect overnight, that isn't a reason to try something new. The main reason to change a product should be if it's causing redness, itchiness, pain, or irritation—not just boredom. Many people get impatient because they don't have realistic expectations for their products, and they switch them for another and expose themselves to a new group of chemicals, setting themselves up for problems.

Q: What kind of moisturizer do I use if I have sensitive skin *and* acne?

A: Number one, simplify. Get back to the basics and detox from any skin care products you don't need (except sunscreen), and let your body find its natural balance. After a month of detox your persistent skin issues will be easier to diagnose by a process of elimination. Your acne might have cleared up or your skin sensitivity lessened because you're not using so many products. Once you identify whether you have sensitive skin or an acne condition or both, begin to investigate why your skin is sensitive or why you may be getting acne. Perhaps you are using drying and irritating acne products to tackle a few pimples and it's given you a sensitive skin condition. Or maybe you have premenstrual acne that comes and goes. I recommend that everyone with acne see a dermatologist before administering any kind of self-treatment. Acne conditions are not created equal, and you may choose (or probably have chosen) the wrong types of products for your particular problem.

When it comes to your three essentials and treating your skin, sensitivity trumps acne. The best products for sensitive skin are not going to make your acne worse, and they will probably help the problem. Try using a gentle lotion cleanser (stay away from the salicylic acid acne washes), and use a water-based lotion to moisturize. It's probably best for you to avoid heavy emollients in your moisturizer, so look for something noncomedogenic that won't clog your pores but that contains water-binding humectants that will keep your sensitive skin hydrated. As with any sensitive skin program, look for products that contain anti-inflammatory ingredients such as allantoin and oatmeal that will help calm down both of your skin issues. Again, don't skip sunscreen. A mineral block like titanium dioxide or zinc oxide may be a better and less irritating than a chemical sunscreen.

>>> skin lie: Wearing facial moisturizer every day and night prevents the development of fine lines.

>>> skin truth: How many times have you heard or read the claim "Minimizes the appearance of fine lines"? Well, that promise is true. A plain old moisturizer containing humectants and emollients will surely fill in fine lines and create a smoother texture. (Notice it the next time you apply any lotion or cream—fine lines do really seem to soften instantly, simply by the act of hydrating the surface of the skin.) Unfortunately, like a magic illusion, that positive superficial effect washes away once the moisturizer is rinsed off. A good, basic moisturizer—one that doesn't contain active ingredients—will help prevent water loss from your skin, build a stronger epidermal barrier, and diminish fine lines temporarily while it's on your face. But studies have not shown that those who moisturize regularly necessarily have fewer wrinkles.

A better question is: Does someone who wears sun protection regularly develop fewer lines? Sun damage causes most wrinkling in the first place. Antioxidants like green tea are currently being studied for their potential to avert free-radical damage and consequently help prevent wrinkles. However, the jury is still out and many antioxidant products don't offer a stable, and thereby effective, form of the ingredient. They also can't substitute for the powerful protection of a sunblock. It's the one proven, preemptive, anti-aging product out there. The only topical skin care products that can truly prevent wrinkling are sunblock and retinoic acid. The regular use of prescription-strength Retin-A has been proven to decrease the development of fine lines and increase the formation of collagen, but this is far different from applying a basic moisturizer every day.

Body Cleansers and Moisturizers

Don't give short shrift to your skin from the neck down. Unless it is sun-exposed, it needs just two daily essentials: soap and moisturizer. Some bar soaps have stronger detergents than others or higher concentrations of surfactants. All of them, including liquid body washes, include at least one surfactant, preservatives, emulsifiers, moisturizing agents, and probably a fragrance. If you have sensitive skin (if you have eczema or psoriasis, for instance), you should avoid synthetic fragrances and harsh detergents. Stay away from antibacterial or deodorant soaps too, since your skin may be intolerant to the added chemicals in them.

Antibacterial soaps are very effective in fighting folliculitis or back acne, but they are extremely drying. You might want to use it every other day. To cleanse dry skin, remember that liquid soaps aren't necessarily gentler or more moisturizing. Liquid is simply the vehicle. Some bar soaps provide the waxy emollients your skin needs to prevent more flaking and dryness. Look for the same emollient ingredients that would be present in a rich facial moisturizer.

The density of pores (and oil glands) is different on the body, so the skin there tends to be dryer. Oil glands are more concentrated on the upper body, which is why you may notice that your legs get especially dry. A lighter body lotion (one with humectants such as glycerin or sodium PCA) is just fine for most of your body, but you may want to use a thicker cream or ointment (with emollients such as squalene and shea butter) for particularly rough, parched parts: hands, feet, elbows, knees, and shins.

It really is true that the sooner you apply body moisturizer after bathing, the more effective it will be. If your skin is still slightly damp, the humectants can retain that moisture while the emollients seal it on. You don't have to play beat the clock after your shower, but this actually does make moisturizing more effective. You should also adjust your body moisturizer in the same way that you tweak your facial routine, depending on how your skin feels. Use a thicker moisturizer in the dry winter if your skin is looking flaky or feeling tight; skip moisturizer on parts of your body that feel fine without it (such as your torso or back).

Your Daily Sunscreen

These days it's so easy to incorporate sunscreen into your daily routine that there's no excuse not to wear it (at least from the collarbone up) every single day. It's difficult to find a daily moisturizer without an SPF, or sun protection factor, of at least 15. Granted, it is incredibly confusing to know what kind of sun protection product to use (Do you need sunblock or sunscreen? SPF 15 or 50?), but one thing is clear: your daily moisturizer must contain sunscreen or sunblock, and you must wear it. If the fear of skin cancer isn't enough, consider that researchers estimate that UV exposure accounts for 80 percent of the skin's aging process (sun spots, wrinkles, dry skin). In a recent survey of more than one thousand American women, more than a third believed the sun to be the number one most negative photoaging factor. But only 45 percent say they wear SPF daily to fight the signs of aging, while more than 50 percent reported using antiaging products to correct those signs. That's like closing the barn door after the horse has escaped—it's too late. The best prevention against photoaging is wearing sunscreen every day. It is the most powerful antiaging product on the market bar none.

SUN OPTIMISM

Too frequently my patients tell me that they like a certain sunscreen, and I ask, "Great, are you wearing it right now?" They usually answer something like, "No, I didn't put sunscreen on today. I was just coming here, and then I'm going back to work." Just going to my office probably amounted to twenty minutes of sun exposure. Just because you're not baking yourself on the beach, it doesn't mean you're not getting sun—and sun damage. UV rays pass through the ozone layer of the atmosphere, and up to 80 percent can come through clouds or pollution too. And they reflect off concrete, just as they reflect off the sand and water at the beach. UVA wavelengths also penetrate windows, so if you're spending time near one (at a restaurant, in your office, in your car, or on a plane), your DNA is getting fried. And UV rays penetrate about two feet into the water, so if you are in the pool or in the ocean, your legs are getting sun.

Of course, the sun is more intense and more dangerous in the summertime, at higher altitudes, in places closer to the equator, and when it directly hits your skin for an extended period of time. But please don't fool yourself into thinking you are safe just because you're in the city (not at the pool), running a quick errand, or driving in your car. Many scientific studies have shown that drivers in the United States who spend a lot of time behind the wheel have an increase of skin cancers and sun damage on their left side (the one nearest the window) due to repeated, cumulative sun exposure. In countries such as England, where the steering wheel is on the opposite side, there are more incidences of skin cancer on the right side.

I think many of us are sun optimists, making excuses (that almost make sense) for not putting on sunblock every day. I hear it all the time. "It's too early in the morning to bother with sunscreen when I go running." "Come on, it's dark and cloudy today, do I really need sunscreen?" "I'm just taking the kids to school, I'll only be outside for a few minutes." Take it seriously. Remember, UV rays are like a laser gun, ready to destroy your DNA the minute you step outside. It's not hard to do, it's not a huge hassle, and with so many different high-tech formulas on the market, it doesn't have to be sticky or greasy either. No more excuses, just do it. Try!

SUNBLOCK VERSUS SUNSCREEN

We throw the two terms around with abandon, but sunblocks and sunscreens are not interchangeable and are not created equal. It's important to realize that most sunscreens (especially the SPF 15 tinted moisturizers or face lotions you would wear every day) don't contain the blocking ingredients that protect against UVA rays, the ones that cause skin cancers and premature aging. Longer UVA wavelengths penetrate to the dermis, where they trigger the melanocytes, creating a suntan (again, a sign that your body has been injured). Many sunscreens safeguard the skin only from UVB rays, which also cause skin cancers and generate sunburns on the surface of the skin: In fact, the SPF factor on a label only gauges protection from UVB rays. You should be aware that there are shorter and longer UVA rays too. (See the "Common Sun Protection Ingredients" table on page 82 to learn which substances filter which wavelengths best.)

To be on the safest side every day, always wear a combination sunblock and sunscreen. It will have "broad spectrum" on the label, which means you'll be getting both UVA and UVB protection. Ideally, you should be on guard against both, and against longer UVA wavelengths too. (In the next chapter, I'll discuss how to protect your skin even more when you're in direct sun—on a beach vacation, at the pool, enjoying outdoor sports, or protecting your children's skin when they're outside playing.)

PHYSICAL SUNBLOCKS

Sunblocks are just that, physical blockers that sit on the skin like armor. UVA and UVB rays ricochet off of sunblock like darts hitting a shield. Titanium dioxide and zinc oxide are the classic mineral sunblocking ingredients. In most products they are micronized, so the tiny nanoparticles are more transparent and less opaque and pasty on your skin. (Remember the chalky white zinc oxide on lifeguards' noses in the old days?) Also, because they are literally mineral, rather than chemical ingredients, they tend to be much less irritating to sensitive skin. Likewise, you could absolutely consider the right kind of clothing, sunglasses, a wide-brimmed hat, and an umbrella to be a type of physical blocker too.

CHEMICAL SUNSCREENS

These are chemical ingredients that filter either UVB or UVA radiation. Instead of creating a physical block that deflects ultraviolet rays, they absorb the sun's light energy and convert it safely into thermal (heat) energy on top of the skin, which is then released. (It sounds like some kind of science fiction magic trick, doesn't it?) A primary scientific premise is that "energy is constant." It can be changed into different forms, like vapor changing to water, then changing to ice, but it's never really gone. So chemical sunscreens don't absorb the UV radiation as much as convert it into something benign (heat) that dissipates from the surface of your skin before it's able to reach the collagen in the dermis and the DNA in your cells. Chemical filters intercept that radiation and transform it into something much less dangerous.

The problem is that this photochemical reaction uses up sunscreen. Imagine that each chemical sunscreen molecule gets zapped and disappears the second it gets hit by a photon and converts to heat. Rather than wearing off, it is actually used up, like gasoline used by a car or food consumed by your body. That's why it must be reapplied. The more sun you are getting, the faster sunscreen is used up or breaks down.

It's also important to realize that chemical UVA blockers are not created equal. Though physical, mineral blockers literally shield skin from both short and long UVA wavelengths, most chemical alternatives aren't able to protect from the entire UVA spectrum. Most protect from the shortwave UVA range. Avobenzone (Parsol 1789) is the only chemical UVA block that prevents long-wave UVA rays from penetrating. But avobenzone is not photostable, so it requires a photostabilizer (such as the new Helioplex) to prevent it from degrading quickly (usually in less than two hours) in sunlight.

The differences among all these polysyllabic active ingredients are confounding but important to comprehend. Some are more protective than others, some absorb only a certain length of UVA ray, and many chemical sunscreens absorb only UVB radiation. Here is a primer so you'll know what to look for and exactly what you're getting protection-wise when you buy a sunscreen or sunblock.

COMMON SUN PROTECTION INGREDIENTS

UVB PROTECTION	UVA PROTECTION	UVB AND UVA PROTECTION
Octinoxate (octyl methoxycinnamate) **Homosalate** **Octisalate** **Para-aminobenzoic acid** (otherwise known as PABA; because it is a skin irritant, most sunscreens are PABA-free) **Octocrylene**	**Avobenzone (Parsol 1789)**, the only chemical that protects against the entire UVA spectrum (long and short rays), but it needs an added photostabilizer (such as Helioplex) to prevent breakdown in the sun. **Mexoryl SX** (Ecamsule) (protects against long and short UVA wavelengths) **Oxybenzone** (for shorter-wave UVA protection)	**Physical sunblocks** (these provide both long and short-wave protection): **Titanium dioxide** **Zinc oxide**

So what kind of ingredients do you need for everyday protection? In general, look for a broad-spectrum product that protects against both UVA and UVB radiation. (UVC wavelengths are much shorter, and don't penetrate the atmosphere.) A facial lotion that contains one or two chemical sunscreens and at least one sunblock (titanium dioxide or zinc oxide) is perfectly adequate. Personally, I always have a few sun protection options available (one for every day, another for exercise, and one with a higher SPF for weekends if I'm outdoors or at the beach). Most days, on my face, I use Aveeno Active Naturals Positively Radiant Daily Moisturizer, SPF 30, which contains chemical UVA and UVB sunscreens. When I exercise outside, I choose something like Coppertone Sport Sunblock Lotion, SPF 30, because it's more adhesive and stays on if I'm sweating. I also like its kids' water-resistant formulation (Coppertone Kids Sunscreen Lotion, SPF 50) because it tends not to sting if it gets in my eyes. And I keep St. Ives Elements Protective Cleanser with SPF 10 in the shower and use it in the morning. It's a good idea for men, like my own husband, who are in sunscreen denial. At least he'll get *some* sun protection with this, which is better than none at all. For the beach, I use Neutrogena Fresh Cooling Body Mist, SPF 45, because it's transparent and easy to apply all over the body (even one's own back). I also love Nia 24 sunscreen because it feels so silky. Buy an assortment of products: lotions, gels, sticks, sprays, hand wipes, and the baby tear free formulations to use around your eyes. Put these various sunscreens in your bathroom, purse, glove compartment, tennis or golf bag, gym locker, and in your desk drawer at the office. The more you see them, the more you'll remember to use them!

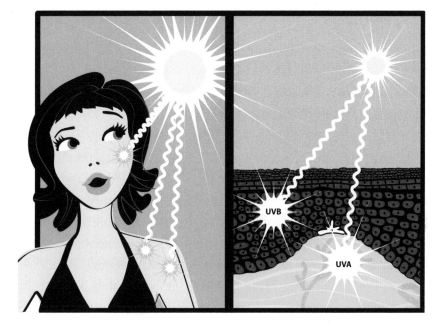

Ultraviolet rays zap your skin at different depths.
UVB damages the epidermis and UVA strikes deeper in the dermis.

SUNSCREEN FORMULATIONS

Why are most sun protection products so greasy and sticky? The gummy, inelegant sunblocks and sunscreens you're thinking about are probably the formulas best suited for a day at the beach. First of all, a higher concentration of active sun-blocking and -screening substances tends to make the solution tackier. Plus, these sunscreens are meant to stay on your skin and not come off, so they have to be adhesive. They include lots of "silicone polymers" and "acrylate polymers," which make them more water-resistant but also stickier on your skin. Acrylate polymer substances are rubbery fixatives, also found in hair sprays, that allow a sunscreen to hold up to water, sweat, and rubbing, but they work by forming a film on your skin. So by all means, for everyday wear, avoid products with terminology like this on the label: "waterproof," "water-resistant," "sweatproof," "sport."

New technology has made sunscreen application less of a hassle. A couple years ago, fine mist sprays began to allow you to apply sunscreen to your own back and help you get it on your kids' skin as you chased them around. The newest delivery system called wash-on uses encapsulated active sunscreen ingredients in a cleanser (like the one I have in the shower). Because the sunscreen is positively charged, it has a magnetic attraction to the skin (which has a natural negative charge), so the active ingredients cling to your face and stay there. Right now, the products provide an SPF of only up to 15, so they aren't enough for a day at the beach. But this could be an easier way to incorporate sun protection into a daily routine, especially if you have oily skin and like to wash it in the morning. Because it's not a lotion or cream, this innovative formulation doesn't leave a sticky, greasy residue.

It's good news that there are so many elegant, lightweight textures of facial lotion with SPF that don't feel too greasy at all. The same rules that pertain to moisturizer formulations apply here. Note that even if you have drier skin, you may find that SPF moisturizers are already hydrating enough since the ingredients needed (in the delivery system) to suspend active sunscreens are silicones and other slippery substances. If you tend to be extremely dry, you can use a cream or lotion containing a humectant such as glycerin or an antioxidant emollient such as tocopherol acetate (vitamin E). For oily skin, go with a gel, spray, or lotion with a high water or alcohol content that will evaporate quickly from your skin, try one of the new SPF cleansers, or use a mineral suncreen powder. Look for "oil-free," "hypoallergenic," and "noncomedogenic" on labels. Those with sensitive skin should try a water-based lotion with physical UVA blockers, since chemical sunscreens often irritate their skin. Blue Lizard is a favorite brand for people with extremely sensitive skin.

>>> q&a

Q: I'm worried about nanoparticles of titanium dioxide and zinc oxide. I heard they can be dangerous. Are they?

A: They could possibly prove harmful because their tiny size may be able to penetrate into the dermis through hair follicles and then into the bloodstream. The good news is that zinc oxide and titanium dioxide used to look like white diaper cream on your skin, and now they've become nearly transparent thanks to this micronization. A lot of mineral makeup and powder sunscreen formulations utilize nanoparticles of titanium dioxide and zinc oxide too. But now this active ingredient, or drug, is not only blocking ultraviolet light by sitting on top of the skin, it's being delivered through the pores into the body. Most sunblocks use nanoparticles (although products don't have to disclose that information on the label). So how microscopic is a nanoparticle? A measurement of a nanometer is one billionth of a meter—approximately one ten-thousandth the diameter of a strand of human hair.

The concern is that these ingredients, if they are absorbed, could then create free radicals that damage DNA. In fairness, the lab studies involving nano-size titanium dioxide didn't concern sunscreens but were done using photoactive titanium dioxide (sun enhancers that break down chemical contamination). Sunscreen products use coated nanoparticles designed to deflect sunlight and are not made to generate free radicals. Most of the scientific studies done on nanoparticles over the past ten years have *not* detected penetration through human skin. Environmental groups such as Friends of the Earth complain that there have not been enough studies done and that products containing nanoparticles should be required to state that on the label. And that's a good point. The Environmental Working Group (EWG), a consumer advocacy organization, still recommends products with these physical blockers, whether they are nano-size or not. They argue that nanoparticles of titanium dioxide and zinc oxide are just as toxic as chemical sunscreens such as oxybenzone and octinoxate that the EWG claims can be absorbed into the skin and cause abnormal activity in the body. For now, I believe the health risk of developing skin cancer from not wearing sunscreen definitely outweighs the danger of using sunblocks containing nanoparticles at least for adults. For babies and children under ten, I would try to avoid nanoparticles.

Q: Do I really need to wear a sunscreen every day on my body, even if I'm not in the sun very much? Is a body lotion with SPF 15 as effective as my beach sunblock?

A: Yes, wear it. But it depends on where you live, what clothes you're wearing, and how long you'll be outside. Your Fitzpatrick Skin Type—how fair or dark your skin is—should also be a clue as to how much protection you need. If you're in Miami in the middle of summer and you're outdoors a lot, you'll need a stronger sunblock, applied over more of your exposed body, than someone wearing a suit in New York City on a cloudy fall day. If it's bright and sunny and you're outside for more than a few minutes, wear a sunblock on exposed areas of skin (including hands, ears, neck, chest, arms, and legs). Unless you're in direct sun all day long, you probably don't need to worry about reapplying sunblock on your body, but do put it on before you go out. Don't overthink it or rationalize that you might not need it. Remember, the sun's rays are killer laser beams. If they're going to be hitting you, protect your skin with the sunblock.

It's mandatory to apply a sunscreen every single day—no matter what—on your face, neck, ears, and upper chest (if it's visible). If most of your body is covered with clothing (which usually has an SPF of less than 10) and you spend much of your time inside, it's not necessary to apply sunscreen head to toe every day—although if you like a particular body lotion with sunscreen, by all means wear it every day. (I use Eucerin Everyday Protection Body Lotion, SPF 15, all the time, and the fact that it has sun protection happens to be an added plus.) And use a hand cream with added sunscreen while you're at it, to help prevent the wrinkling and sun spots that are telltale signs of your age. (Most women's hands, chests, and shoulders look years older than their faces, just because they neglect to protect and moisturize them.)

A broad-spectrum body lotion with an SPF of 15 is better than nothing but not as protective as the broad-spectrum sunblock (with the harder-core sunscreens and blockers) that you might wear poolside. Most daily moisturizers with SPF add one or two chemical sunscreens and maybe one chemical UVA blocker (remember that SPF only measures protection from UVB rays). Usually that chemical sunscreen is benzophone 3 or oxybenzone, which guards only against short UVA wavelengths. If you're going to be spending time in direct sunlight (not just a day at the beach but a ride in a convertible or lunch at an outdoor café), opt for a broad-spectrum product that contains chemical UVB absorbers and either physical blockers (titanium dioxide or zinc oxide) or chemical UVA protectors like Mexoryl or avobenzone that prevent longer wavelengths from reaching the dermis.

>>> skin lie: A sunscreen with SPF 50 blocks 50 percent of the sun's rays.

>>> skin truth: How I wish this were true. Unfortunately, it's incorrect on more than one count. First, as SPF measures a product's ability to protect the skin only from UVB rays, that's only half the story. It quantifies the amount of time you can be in the sun wearing sunscreen before you are burned. So if you are fair-skinned and would begin to burn in ten minutes without sun protection, wearing an SPF of 15 will protect you fifteen times as long—for 150 minutes (10 x 15 = 150). Confusing, right? SPF math is also deceptive because the numbers don't add up. SPF 30 does not double the protection of SPF 15, for example. It would figure that you should be able to stay in the sun thirty times longer, but that's not the case. An SPF 15 allegedly blocks 93 to 95 percent of UVB rays, while an SPF 30 supplies 97 percent coverage. So bumping your SPF to over 50 doesn't make it that much more protective. It may be advantageous to check the percentages of active ingredients on the back of the label, in addition to the SPF number on the front. One top brand increases the amount of active ingredients, almost doubling the percentage of some, from an SPF 45 sunblock to an SPF 55. Those numbers do add up, especially since both products contain UVA filters too. Don't let SPF numbers give you a false sense of security. It's more important to look for "broad-spectrum" UVA and UVB protection and check exactly how much of the active ingredients you're getting from one sunscreen to another.

Also, don't assume that applying an SPF 15 tinted moisturizer over an SPF 15 facial lotion will magically turn into SPF 30. You still have on SPF 15. Imagine two stereo speakers; one is set to volume 5 and another is set at volume 5. You're not at volume level 10. However, because you're doubling the amount of SPF product, you are probably getting more protection, just by virtue of the quantity you're applying. When sunscreens are tested, they are applied as thick as icing to get that SPF rating. We usually don't put on a thick coat of sunscreen, so we're getting only a fraction of the protection we think we are. When you use an SPF 15 on your face, you usually rub on a very thin layer and the SPF probably drops down to 5 or less. So doubling up your SPF won't hurt, although it won't add up to twice as much protection either. Bottom line: buy sunblock/sunscreen SPF 55 or less, and reapply every hour when outside in the sun.

>>> q&a

Q: I wear a tinted moisturizer with SPF 20. Is that enough for every day?

A: It's better than nothing but not as effective as wearing a translucent facial lotion with sunscreen. Why? Most of us desire a natural, less-is-more look with our makeup, and less is not more when it comes to sun protection. Applying a sheer layer of tinted moisturizer or a dusting of mineral makeup gives you a fraction of the SPF you thought you were getting. Unless your makeup application is spackled on, you're not getting enough sunscreen from your makeup. It's better to think of SPF makeup as a booster for your daily sunscreen/moisturizer. Apply it on top of your SPF moisturizer. And mineral powder foundation, which contains natural titanium dioxide and zinc oxide, is a brilliant way to reapply your sunscreen during the day and touch up your makeup at the same time.

Q: Can I use my wife's skin care products?

A: Please do! I wish my husband would steal my skin care stash, especially my sunscreen. Male skin is totally different from female skin on some levels and exactly the same on others. Your hormones tend to produce more oil on your face than women's do. But if you shave every day, that exfoliates the skin, which can lead to dryness. And using shaving cream, which is a form of soap, may dry it out even more. If it does, use a light moisturizer. One thing you can probably skip is a facial wash, since rinsing your skin in the shower is probably sufficient. Do you need your own special line of men's products? Not really.

It's a matter of personal preference, since they're essentially all the same ingredients—just wrapped up in more masculine packaging. If the scent of one of your wife's moisturizers is too girly, go for a more unisex, fragrance-free type. You should also have your own product at the ready to treat ingrown hairs that may get inflamed or irritation from shaving (something like Bliss Ingrown Hair Eliminating Peeling Pads with salicylic acid to keep pores unplugged and moisturizing glycerin to soothe the skin).

Most important—I'll repeat it again—every single man, woman, and child must wear a sunscreen daily. That includes when you are going to the office or driving in a car, not just playing tennis or running in the park. In a recent consumer poll done by the American Academy of Dermatology, 65 percent of men said they used sunscreen when outdoors. However, only 5 percent use sunscreen on a daily basis—which may be why skin cancer is the number one cancer in men over the age of fifty, ahead of prostate, lung, and colon cancer. Not good enough, guys. If you have to snag your wife's sunscreen, go ahead. Just do it every day.

Q: How do I need to adjust my daily regimen for my dark (African-American) skin?

A: The biggest challenge of darker skin is pigmentation problems. When your skin is irritated, by either scrubbing too hard or picking at a pimple, it can easily become discolored. Any form of trauma, even a small scratch or redness, can turn into a dark stain that lasts for about six months. To help fade darker spots, ask your dermatologist about including either hydroquinone (a lightening agent) or retinoic acid in your regimen. As for your routine, keep it geared to how your skin feels (oily or dry), but if there's any confusion, it's most likely sensitive. If your skin is pigmentation-prone, it is definitely very sensitive. You want to avoid anything that will cause a reaction on the skin: fragrances, exfoliants that are too gritty, acids that are too strong, and benzoyl peroxide acne treatments. Even a harsh cleanser can cause pigmentation problems. Start by using gentle products that contain anti-inflammatory ingredients such as aloe vera, allantoin, soy, vitamin E, and cucumber. And you need to wear sunscreen daily to prevent more hyperpigmentation. Even though your skin type is a little more protected by melanin, it's not completely safe from skin cancer or burning. Sun exposure generates skin tone discoloration, and those darker spots are hypersensitive to the sun, so sunscreen is important. Remember, don't pick or scratch your face, which can cause dark spots. You have to be especially respectful of, and gentle to, this type of skin.

Three Extras: Options to Have at the Ready

I mentioned that your medicine chest should be stocked with a mighty (but tiny) arsenal of well-chosen products that you can draw on if you need them. You won't use them every day, but I've found, personally and professionally, that these three items are always good to have around.

An Exfoliant

By the time I reached the age of thirty, I had an epiphany about exfoliating my skin. It made all the difference. Sloughing off of dead skin cells instantly brightens a complexion and makes it look and feel fresher. It smoothes the texture, improves skin tone, and helps unclog pores, all at the same time. Dead keratinocytes are opaque, so light flattens against them. They're like dirt on a windshield.

Though including some kind of exfoliant in your weekly routine is beneficial, overexfoliating is dangerous. Make sure you use only one exfoliating option—an AHA cleanser used once or twice a week or an AHA lotion once or twice a week, but not both. If you use a facial scrub weekly, you don't need a glycolic acid product too.

Exfoliation, the process of stripping off the top layer of skin, is absolutely necessary for someone who has acne or who complains of rough, dull skin. The question is, which exfoliating method should you use? A chemical exfoliant is an acid that interacts with the dead cells to get rid of them, while a mechanical exfoliant scrubs them off physically. Most of us can use either one of these methods, and often a product will employ both (a sugar and fruit enzyme scrub, for example). There are also at-home versions of more powerful, doctor's office procedures, such as chemical peels and microdermabrasion. I'll address the professional-strength techniques in chapter 10, but the do-it-yourself kinds are easy, effective, and safe because they are much milder. The FDA prohibits a consumer product from having more than 10% AHA concentration, while doctors can use much higher concentrations, such as 50%.

CHEMICAL EXFOLIATION

Acid-based exfoliants interact immediately with the skin and dissolve dead cells. These utilize beta-hydroxy acid (or salicylic acid) and alpha-hydroxy acids. Under the AHA banner are glycolic acid (derived from sugarcane), citric acid, lactic acid (from milk), and fruit enzymes. Whether in the form of a gel, cream, lotion, or even a cleanser, all of these chemicals basically produce a slight chemical peel. That's why many products are labeled "peel treatment," "retexturizing peel," or "peel pads," (acid-soaked pads that you swipe over your face, then follow with another neutralizing pad containing moisturizing ingredients).

Salicylic acid is definitely the exfoliant of choice for someone with oily or acne-prone skin. Because, unlike AHAs, salicylic acid is oil-soluble, it's able to unglue a keratin plug and penetrate through the sebum to the lining of the pore, releasing some of the oil and bacteria before it can cause acne. It also has anti-inflammatory properties (since it's derived from a compound similar to aspirin).

For someone with very dry or sensitive skin, lactic acid is the best and gentlest option (see the Q&A on page 94), since citric, fruit, and glycolic acids can be too harsh. But read the label carefully. Sometimes a product contains many different kinds of acids, which together can be far too strong. (I counted six in one over-the-counter exfoliant alone!) As a general rule, if a product contains more than three acid substances, it could potentially be irritating.

MECHANICAL EXFOLIATION

As old school as it sounds, this method involves physically scrubbing the dead skin off your face. The means can be as elementary as a washcloth or soft brush. A product uses a gritty, granular substance, suspended in a cream, lotion, or gel, that manually scrubs off the surface layer. Granules such as oatmeal, polyethylene beads, salt, sugar, calcium carbonate, dimethicone polymers, or tiny crystal particles are used as gentle buffing tools. Do-it-yourself microdermabrasion kits use a "resurfacing tool" (sounds scary, but it's just a slightly abrasive sponge or soft-bristle brush) to massage a cream with aluminum oxide or mineral crystals onto the skin. If you have a tendency toward sensitivity or rosacea, too much abrasive scrubbing can irritate your skin. It is better to stick with a super-gentle lactic acid exfoliant and use it only once or twice a month at most.

HOW TO EXFOLIATE SAFELY, AND HOW OFTEN TO DO IT

Whether you use a chemical or mechanical exfoliant or one that incorporates both, be careful to apply it for only a short time. An acid works immediately, so it doesn't need to be on your face for more than three or four minutes. Wash it off right away if it hurts or stings (it should create a tingling sensation, not any kind of burning pain). Even if they're made from natural fruit acids, these are still strong chemicals and can injure the skin to the point of causing erosion and even scarring. By the same token, scrubbing too hard or too long (more than one minute) with a mechanical exfoliant can literally rub skin raw. Be extra-gentle on the softer parts of your face (the neck and cheeks especially). You could break blood vessels and scratch the skin. Don't forget: when you exfoliate—or cleanse or moisturize—always include your neck and the upper chest. Treat those areas as part of your face.

Exfoliating too often is yet another example of overdoing a good thing. Like everything else, moderation is golden. Only oily or acne-prone skin should be exfoliated more than twice a week. If you have sensitive or dry skin, once or twice a month is sufficient, and more than that could be detrimental. I find that people don't always know the purpose of the products they are using or the ingredients they contain. This can lead to an overload of more than one exfoliating ingredient in your regimen, which can lead to irritation. With all but the oiliest skin, it's extremely important to moisturize after you scrub or use an acid exfoliant. Your skin has been stripped of its uppermost layer and needs that moisture and protective barrier replenished. For the same reason, it's vital to apply sunscreen when you use exfoliants—AHAs have been shown to increase sun sensitivity by 50 percent. You want to protect that fresh, beautiful skin you've just uncovered. Exfoliation will make your skin more sensitive to anything you apply to it: sunscreens, moisturizers, perfumes, or medicines.

>>> q&a

Q: My skin is dry and sensitive, and exfoliating seems to make my rosacea worse. Is there an alternative to harsh acids or scrubs?

A: Scrubbing can aggravate rosacea or a painfully dry complexion. And because acids work by temporarily lowering the natural pH balance of the skin, they can be very irritating for someone with sensitivity. The gentlest option is lactic acid, which is probably the cheapest and easiest exfoliant around. Just soak a washcloth in plain whole milk, then rest the damp cloth on your face, neck, and upper chest for a minute or two. (You can dunk the cloth again and repeat, but don't overdo it and cause inflammation. Four minutes on your skin is more than enough to see results.) Essentially, you're getting a light chemical peel, but the fatty proteins in the milk act as a moisturizing buffer to the lactic acid. Milk also has anti-inflammatory and humectant properties that help to soothe and moisturize skin simultaneously. Talk about a perfect (and organic) beauty food!

Q: Is a body scrub something I need to use in the shower once a week?

A: "Need" is the key word here. A body scrub can feel luxurious, smell delicious, and leave your skin smooth and moisturized. But in all honesty, a nubby washcloth and soap do just as well at exfoliating and cleansing. (I like to use a more abrasive loofah for ankles, feet, hands, and elbows.) Often body scrubs contain both mechanical and chemical exfoliants, and because they are meant to work on tougher skin (not on your face or neck), they may be severe or irritating (most are quite oily too). If you have a scratch or any irritation, or even if you've just shaved your legs, a body scrub (especially one with fruit enzymes or acids) can burn or sting like crazy. If you want to use a scrub, don't rub it on too aggressively, and use it no more than once a week. Even if your skin can tolerate it initially, scrubbing too often can eventually leave it inflamed.

If you have eczema, stay away from abrasive exfoliants and any kind of acid. They can make the problem much worse. You really need an emollient-rich moisturizer instead of a scrub. For someone with psoriasis, especially if it has formed a dry, silvery layer, try a cream or lotion containing salicylic or lactic acid. This creamy acid formula will help dissolve that thick surface more gently than a scratchy mechanical scrub. Plus, this allows emollients to get through that heavy scale. As with any exfoliant, once or twice a week is plenty. Exfoliant abuse can absolutely damage the skin's barrier function. It can actually create new psoriasis by traumatizing the skin, a phenomenon called koebnerization.

A Benzoyl Peroxide Spot Treatment

It's inevitable: we're all going to wake up with a pimple (or a few) occasionally. It's smart to be prepared with a good acne-fighting solution. Combined with a salicylic acid exfoliant (whether it be a cleanser, a liquid, or a lotion), benzoyl peroxide makes up the second part of a one-two punch against pimples. A topical benzoyl peroxide treatment (usually in the form of a gel or liquid) will kill the bacteria that are causing the breakout, help unclog the offending pore, and reduce inflammation, whereas salicylic acid only unplugs the pore. Over-the-counter strengths of benzoyl peroxide usually range from 2.5% to 10%, and I think 5% and up works most effectively. Higher concentrations are available by prescription but risk irritating and drying the skin. Benzoyl peroxide can help to prevent acne flare-ups before they come to a head, so to speak, so the best time to apply it is in the early stage, when the bump is little and hasn't yet erupted. If you always break out in a particular area, you can apply the product there regularly. In fact, a 2004 study published in *The Lancet* found that topical benzoyl peroxide treatments are as effective as taking prescription oral antibiotics for some cases of acne.

A Topical Steroid Cream

Another foreseeable skin emergency (for you or someone else in your family) is a rash, itchiness, or red, irritated skin. Every family should have 1% hydrocortisone cream in the medicine cabinet just in case. If this over-the-counter, low-dose product isn't effective (and it's often not as fast or successful an antidote as you might need), get a prescription-strength version from your dermatologist. It's fantastic for treating a burn (even a sunburn) or any kind of irritation on the skin. You need to have something immediate that you can put on, just like taking aspirin when you have a headache. This is a great antidote for eczema, bug bites, and allergic contact dermatitis (as from poison ivy). But if used on normal, nonrashy skin, topical steroids can lead to stretch marks, so they should only be used temporarily (for a maximum of two weeks).

Unnecessary Luxuries: Products You Don't Need (but Love!)

They sure are fun to buy and lovely to use, and all the jars and bottles look pretty in your bathroom, but these cosmetic options are far from essential. If they're not in your budget and you don't have the time for a twenty-minute face mask or an added step in your nightly regimen, then skip them—and don't feel guilty about it. When it comes to cleansing, moisturizing, and protecting, these three things won't do anything more for your skin than your three essentials. If you want to treat yourself to a special skin care purchase or an at-home facial, go for it. I don't blame you, and I do it too. But please don't be tricked into thinking you need it.

Eye Cream

If you're going to cancel one item from your shopping list, this is the one. It's just as effective, and far more efficient, to multitask with your regular moisturizer and daytime SPF. Yes, it feels nice, but, no, it is not a necessity. In actuality, it's simply redundant. The skin around your eyes is more delicate, but unless you are massaging a thick balm on the rest of your face, the moisturizer you use on your face and neck has the same formulation and many of the same ingredients that you get in any eye cream. The same moisturizing ingredients can treat the fine lines and dryness around your eyes just as well as they take care of the same issues anywhere else on your face.

What about puffiness or dark circles? I'll tackle both those issues in chapter 8, "Skin SOS," but suffice it to say that an eye cream isn't going to eliminate them. Dark circles are due primarily to your anatomy, while puffiness is often a sign of water retention inside your body (often from lack of sleep). A cool compress or cold, damp chamomile tea bags will calm puffiness better than a special eye cream, although they are both temporary cures. If you are bothered by puffiness around your eyes, make sure your regular moisturizer contains anti-inflammatory ingredients such as chamomile, cucumber, or aloe vera (which would be found in an eye cream as well).

Toner

In a classic comedy bit, Jerry Seinfield speculates about why women need all those truckloads of cotton balls. How can they possibly use so many, and for what possible purpose? The answer: toner. How many cotton balls and bottles of astringent did we go through in high school and college, anyway? Toner is meant to remove residual makeup and oil from the skin. But since most cleansers these days do that just fine, toner is an unnecessary added step. Gentle, soothing alcohol-free toners (they usually contain moisturizing or anti-inflammatory substances like rosewater or cucumber) are totally superfluous if you use a moisturizer. (However, I do prefer them, even to makeup remover, to take off any extra bits of eye makeup or concealer because the consistency is so watery.) An alcohol-based astringent toner (similar to the antiseptic version we all remember as teenagers) usually contains ingredients such as witch hazel or salicylic acid to get rid of oil. For those who are addicted to washing their faces in the morning, a quick swipe of toner instead may be just the right remedy. These are great for combination skin conditions, to eliminate oil from one area of the face (rather than all over). For the most part, I, like Seinfeld, don't have much use for cotton balls.

Face Masks

I relish the thought of giving myself an at-home facial, relaxing in front of the TV wearing some kind of blue or green face mask. The odds of this happening (with four kids, a crazy schedule, and a husband who would laugh himself silly) are slim to none. But so are the chances that a mask—whether it be one for moisturizing or a clay mask to "soak up" oil—can do something really transformative or long-lasting to my skin. Can a mask super-moisturize your face and seal the hydration in? Yes, but only until it's rinsed off. Truthfully, masks are like ChapStick for your face—an occlusive film over the surface that provides a nice, temporary fix. For someone with sensitive or rosacea skin, a mask packed with anti-inflammatory ingredients (such as aloe vera, allantoin, and chamomile) and humectants will feel wonderful and soothe the skin, but only while it's on the face. Again, it's always important to read the label, especially if your skin is feeling sensitive. Fruit acids or menthol, which are commonly found in masks, could cause irritation.

Moisturizing Masks

If a mask has active ingredients, such as anti-inflammatories or antioxidants, they might be better absorbed into the skin because of the occlusive barrier of the mask. But that's a big "if," since those ingredients would have to be lipophilic (oil-loving and compatible with skin) and microscopic enough to penetrate pores in the first place. By the same principle of occlusion, I sometimes treat eczema on the body by applying a steroid cream, then putting plastic wrap over it to provide an occlusive barrier so the cream doesn't evaporate or wipe off. This also provides a slight pressure that pushes the medication onto the skin. It's similar to slathering on a rich foot cream and then covering the feet with cotton socks—although, unlike a medicine, the moisturizing effect wears off the minute you wash your skin.

Clay Masks

Clay masks don't actually absorb or "soak up" oil, and they can't really "purify" and "detoxify" your pores either. A mask with kaolin (a mineral-rich clay), sea mud, or even charcoal does provide a gentle way of exfoliating by coating the skin like an adhesive. When it dries and is rinsed off, the mask theoretically pulls off some dead cells, debris, and oil with it. It's the same concept as rolling a lint brush over the surface of a sweater. Pore strips work the same way, and they're terrific. Sometimes a clay mask contains active ingredients like sulfur, which is a natural antibacterial and anti-inflammatory, or tea tree oil, a natural antiseptic and anti-inflammatory. But a treatment like this won't be more effective than a salicylic acid exfoliant and diligent nightly cleansing. A clay mask can reduce the oil you have right now, but unfortunately it's just going to build up again in no time.

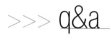 >>> q&a

Q: What about D.I.Y. masks made with avocado, olive oil, or honey? Do those work just as well as store-bought products?

A: They are absolutely as effective. However, in my opinion, 99 percent of the benefit of using either a purchased or a homemade mask is simply the act of washing your face. Putting food on your face can be as effective as a retail product and the food contains natural forms of the same ingredients. You can use a humectant (like honey), an emollient (such as avocado or olive oil), an anti-inflammatory (cucumbers or oatmeal), or a gentle exfoliant (such as milk or yogurt) to achieve the desired outcome. But, just like a store-bought face mask, the results last only as long as the product stays on your face. The honey and avocado aren't penetrating deep into the skin, they're just sitting on top of it for a while. If you prefer to make your own home brew, have fun and go for it. Like any other skin care product, though, do your research and choose the natural components that will be best for the skin you are having that day. But honestly, it might be even more beneficial to simply eat the stuff.

Q: Don't I need a facial once in a while to really deep clean my skin? Are extractions safe?

A: I hate to be the bearer of shocking news, but deep cleaning is a myth and facials are completely unnecessary—although they are wonderfully luxurious. I'm still confused as to why my friends dedicate so much precious money and time to facials. But if they're enjoyable and make you feel better about how you look, I suppose they're worth every penny—but they are not directly medicinal. I recently read a *New York Times* article about expensive and famous facialists in New York City who insist that their clients must get weekly facials (costing something like $500) or run the risk of their skin looking awful and old immediately, and irreversibly. That's just a scare tactic. Don't believe it.

A facial treatment typically consists of cleansing, moisturizing, exfoliating, applying some kind of mask, maybe a light peel (the same concentration you can get over-the-counter), and a facial massage. You can do all the same things yourself at home (granted, without the spa luxury of it all). The massage is probably the part you would leave out in the D.I.Y. version, and it may be the most beneficial and relaxing step, since it gets your blood flow going and brings oxygen and other nourishment to your skin. The downside to all that massage and exfoliating is an anti-inflammatory response that causes some of us to break out. As far as deep cleaning goes, all anyone needs to do is exfoliate—with either a mechanical scrub or an acid—in order to unplug the keratin from the pores and see a dermatologist if you have a chronic condition such as acne.

If you want to get a facial (and again, I love them too), be sure to tell a facialist if you have rosacea or acne, if you are using retinoids or any kind of acid product on your face at home, and if you take any prescription drugs that might cause your skin to be hypersensitive. And do your own quality control: make sure the facialist is licensed, and check to see that all the products, equipment, and surfaces are pristine.

Extractions of active acne (whether it is the pustule type we call a pimple or a comedone, which we refer to as a blackhead) are tricky and unnecessary and can be unsafe too. I don't recommend them. Although extractions seem to miraculously (and sometimes painfully) take away the gunk in your pores, it's basically a manual form of exfoliation (extracting the keratin plug from your pore). Putting so much pressure on the hair follicle (or pore) to pop out the dead keratinocytes squeezes the base of the follicle. In the case of a comedone (a type of acne referred to as a "blackhead" or "whitehead"), this can push the oils and benign bacteria so far down the follicle shaft that they burst out the bottom into your skin tissue. That rupture can cause inflammation and ultimately leave a scar or a cyst on your skin, especially on darker skin types. Often, blackheads on the nose are just hair follicles, so trying to extract something from them is ineffectual and could cause scarring or hyperpigmentation. Dermatologists are trained to look at the skin using a microscope, so we truly see it with X-ray vision. We can tell a whitehead, or comedone, from a benign cyst and a blackhead from a hair follicle. Even the best, most skilled facialist doesn't understand the skin microscopically and isn't a medically trained diagnostician.

Q: Should I steam my skin to open up the pores?

A: Let's just dispel all the myths at once. Deep cleaning doesn't happen, and a pore doesn't open and close like a valve. That being said, steaming your face does increase humidity and the water content of the stratum corneum. The heat dilates blood vessels and brings more circulation to the periphery, and that plumps up the skin. But the pores themselves don't have a response to this, although they may appear to be more "open" because your skin is plumper. As the water evaporates from your skin, they appear to "close" again. A word of caution: hot water vapor so near your skin can scald it, and for someone with rosacea steaming is a recipe for disaster. Although it may sound counterintuitive, the evaporation of the water vapor will dry out your skin poststeaming, so you must use a moisturizer afterward.

Natural and Organic Skin Care: The Butterfly Effect

In 1972, the meteorologist Edward Lorenz developed the "butterfly effect," his chaos theory concerning the behavior of weather systems. He concluded that a tiny change in the atmosphere could set off a chain of events that would create a large-scale phenomenon. In essence, a butterfly flapping its wings in Brazil can set off a tornado in Texas. One seemingly insignificant change halfway around the earth can lead to so much. Right now, we're all trying to make our little contribution to improving our ailing environment—changing to energy-efficient lightbulbs, refusing to use petroleum-based plastic grocery bags—and buying products in biodegradable and recycled containers is just one more helpful butterfly flutter.

More than 11 billion personal care products are sold in the United States each year, so why not choose the ones that are safest for the environment? That's reason enough to use certified organic products: we can have our own small, but mighty, impact on the earth every day as consumers. I admit to feeling quite a bit of green guilt, even though I've led canoeing and camping trips and think of myself as such a nature girl. I've been naive—trusting the government to do the thinking and acting on environmental change for me. I realize that I need to take on more responsibility, so I have to start asking myself: Do my products come in recycled containers? Am I recycling them when I'm done with them? Are the ingredients grown with sustainable agriculture? Are they biodegradable? To me, environmentally conscious manufacturing and packaging is what gives the edge to many natural beauty products, even more than their use of nonsynthetic ingredients. It's so easy to cop out, to question whether one's own little attempt is worth it. Why bother when so many other consumers all over the world are dumping their inorganic packaging in the trash (not the recycling bin), which then ends up in a landfill and takes months, if not hundreds of years, to biodegrade. But if I make my own effort, I feel better, and if other people do too, an entire revolution can begin. Even if saving the planet sounds like a wildly abstract notion, it's not so hard to take baby steps with our beauty products. Yes, it's worth the effort, and your one butterfly flutter counts.

It's clear that a majority of us really want to clean up our acts. According to *Nutrition Business Journal,* U.S. retail sales of natural and organic personal care products were $7.5 billion in 2005 and approached $9 billion at the end of 2007. Americans spent approximately $50 billion on cosmetics and toiletries in 2006, so natural and organic products represent about 15 percent of the total market. Two thousand new "natural" or "organic" personal care products were launched in 2006 (up from the approximately eight hundred that were introduced the previous year), according to the Natural Marketing Institute. In this booming beauty market, it's more important than ever to find out if a product is really natural or organic.

Every other item on the retail shelves seems to have "100% Natural," "Organic," or "Green" on the label, but what does that really signify? A recent survey by Bearing Point, a management and technology consulting firm, found that 71 percent of U.S. companies market the "environmental friendliness" of their products to customers. But another poll (by Ipsos) found that 70 percent of Americans felt that when a company labels a product as "green," it's usually just a marketing tactic. The bottom line: we need to be smart about picking the real thing. Just because something says it's natural or organic, it is not a guarantee of authenticity.

In a survey conducted by *Health Magazine,* 83 percent of consumers polled indicated that they prefer to buy all-natural body products, although more than half of them could not define "natural" or "organic." Join the club! First of all, natural and organic are not synonymous. Often "100% Natural" or "All Natural" is 100 percent bogus. The FDA does not regulate the use of "natural," "botanical," "pure," or "organic," so any company can slap them on any product. This practice is known as greenwashing, or brainwashing consumers into believing products are natural when they actually are not. "Organic" refers to the agricultural method in which the ingredients are farmed without pesticides or chemical fertilizers and utilizing renewable resources to save energy. A product vetted by the USDA as "certified organic" must contain 95 percent organically grown ingredients, but what about the other 5 percent? The truth is, we shouldn't take anything at face value, so we need to look carefully at the label. Are chemical preservatives (such as parabens) listed on the ingredients list? Does the box or label bear a certification seal? Does the packaging state that it's "biodegradable" or "recycled"? I actually go online and do some research too, checking a manufacturer's Web site to see how it makes and packages its products. For example, some companies work actively to recycle, to reduce emissions at their manufacturing plants, and even to use solar and wind power. Many use corn-derived plastic and recycled fiber (such as bamboo and wood pulp) and vegetable-based inks in their packaging materials.

The United States is woefully behind Europe in regulating and certifying the authenticity of natural or organic cosmetics and creating comprehensive national standards in the industry. Organic cosmetic products in Europe are regulated by independent agencies: France's Ecocert, Britain's Soil Association, and BDIH in Germany. You can find their stamp on products available all over the United States as well. Guidelines are just now being instituted and enforced here, propelled by eco-conscious retailers and manufacturers. As in the European model, instead of one overall government-funded agency there are a few trade organizations putting initiatives in place. To keep it straight and to look for the right logos on the labels, look at the following chart. These seals of approval can help you make a smarter choice in the "green" market.

Organic Certifications

These logos ensure a measure of quality and authenticity for organic cosmetics. For example, every Ecocert-certified product is inspected to verify that at least 95 percent of the ingredients are organically derived. The USDA has three divisions, the best being "100% Organic," which means that all the ingredients are organically farmed.

ORGANIZATION	WHAT IS IT?	WEBSITE	WHAT IT LOOKS LIKE	WHAT IT MEANS
U.S. Department of Agriculture's National Organic Program (NOP)	The USDA branch regulating organic agricultural products	www.usda .gov		"100% Organic" requires all ingredients to be organic; "Certified Organic" must be at least 95% organic; "Made with Organic" must be at least 70% organic.
Organic & Sustainable Industry Standards (OASIS)	Health and beauty trade association	www .oasisseal.org		At least 85% of ingredients must be certified organic.
Premium Body Care (Whole Foods Market)	Leading retailer of natural and organic foods	www .wholefoods market.com		Prohibits use of 250 synthetic ingredients (parabens, chemical sunscreens, etc.).
Natural Products Association	Leaders of natural products industry	www.natural products assoc.org		Products must be made up of at least 95% natural ingredients, with no ingredients that pose a health risk. Nonnatural ingredients are allowed only when a natural alternative is unavailable.

ORGANIZATION	WHAT IS IT?	WEBSITE	WHAT IT LOOKS LIKE	WHAT IT MEANS
Ecocert	French organic certification organization	www.ecocert .com		At least 95% of ingredients must have a natural origin: at least 10% of total ingredients must be certified organic.
BDIH	German organic certification organization	www.kontrolli erte-naturko smetik.de/en		Prohibits use of many synthetic substances (silicones, petroleum products, paraffin).
The Soil Association	The United Kingdom's leading charity certification organization for organic food and farming	www.soil association .org		Allows a few preservative chemicals to be used; products must use minimal processing.

Once you've found a few wonderful organic products (and there are many high-quality, chemical-free options to choose from), will that "green" cleanser or moisturizer be as good as a more synthetic product? Yes, indeed. Basic cleansers and moisturizers (ones that don't contain active chemical ingredients such as sunscreens or retinoids) will be just as effective. Though the benefits of going green are obvious (fewer potentially toxic chemicals on your skin, organic and healthy ingredients, feeling good about your little butterfly flutter for the earth), there are a couple negatives that you should know about too. Authentic natural products can have a shorter shelf life because they don't contain chemical preservatives. Also, ingredients can separate or may not have the same texture or scent that you are used to due to the lack of silicone and chemical perfumes. To fill this void naturally, essential oils such as rose, sandalwood, and or jasmine are often added for fragrance, and organic shea butter replaces silicone to provide a smoother feel. Many manufacturers have been forced to come up with lots of creative solutions like that—finding natural alternatives for crucial chemical ingredients. Researchers at one organic brand discovered that soy lecithin, an emulsifier that binds oil and water ingredients together in packaged organic foods works well as a cosmetic emulsifier too.

A disturbing phenomenon associated with naturally derived ingredients (for all kinds of cosmetics, whether they are organic or not) is the destruction of indigenous tree species such as sandalwood and palm because they are being stripped for their extracts. Deforestation of sandalwood forests to attain the perfumed oil isn't exactly a politically correct manufacturing method. Conservation and sustainability should be a prime concern of the manufacturers of natural cosmetics. Go online and find out what kind of preservation a company undertakes and how it cultivates its ingredients. We should not only look after our skin with natural elements but also demand that companies protect the precious resources those ingredients come from. Two useful databases are: www.ewg.org and www.thegoodguide.com.

>>> skin lie: Natural or organic ingredients are less irritating to sensitive skin.

>>> skin truth: Organic cleansers and moisturizers can provide the same results as their synthetic counterparts, and therefore they have the potential to irritate the skin too. Most people don't recognize that natural ingredients are still chemicals. An orange contains vitamin C, which is ascorbic acid. A doctor might say "ascorbic acid," and in the natural beauty world it's known as "vitamin C," but it basically boils down to the same thing. The ingredient tocopherol (used as a conditioning agent in most synthetic products) is a derivative of natural vitamin E. Many soaps, synthetic detergents and organic surfactants are derived from a natural vegetable source (primarily coconuts), so it becomes a question of how that source becomes a cleansing agent. They all started as coconuts after all, but by what chemical processes do they become surfactants?

Botanical elements and pure essential oils such as tea tree oil, menthol, eucalyptus, willow bark (a natural form of salicylic acid), and especially citrus (natural
citric acid) can cause allergies or irritation. Mushroom extract contains kojic acid (a
natural skin lightening agent), and papaya and pumpkin enzymes exfoliate the skin
because they are alpha-hydroxy acids. These elements can sometimes be even
stronger in their natural forms. It's important to test any product, even a natural
one, on the inside of your arm or on your neck before using it on your face. It's a
myth that a product must sting to be effective. That pain is actually an alarm bell.

How to Read a Label

Who actually reads the very, very fine print on the side or back of a box?
The ingredients are so indecipherable that they might as well be written
in another language. But the label is extraordinarily important. It's the
one place to find accurate information about the product, and looking at
the information with a discerning eye will equal empowerment at the
cosmetics counter. You can see that a sunscreen offers a decent percentage of both UVA and UVB sunscreens or that a cleanser contains a harsh
detergent or ingredients that will dry your skin. If the label shows that a
moisturizer includes lots of heavy emollients (such as lanolin, mineral
oil, and shea butter), you know it will be too greasy if you have generally
oily skin. The ingredients listing provides the best guide for finding the
most effective and least irritating products for your particular complexion. You just have to learn to decipher the code.

One reason the organic cosmetics market is booming could be our
growing awareness (and wariness) of certain ingredients, specifically the
fact that some chemicals can be harmful. There's much controversy surrounding synthetic substances such as paraben preservatives that have
been tagged as potentially carcinogenic. And many additives, such as
sulfites (used as preservatives) and silicones, can be irritating or harmful to
the skin. The list below spells it out for you clearly, but keep in mind that
scientific testing may not be entirely conclusive. For instance, when an ingredient is classified as potentially dangerous, that toxicity might occur if it

is ingested in large quantities—but not necessarily when a tiny amount is applied topically. In fact, the chemical may not even have been tested on human skin. For example, propylene glycol is a component of industrial antifreeze when it is at 100 percent concentration. The amount of propylene glycol used in a cosmetic product is infinitesimal in comparison. Sometimes the science needed to strongly back up these scary claims is just not yet available. That being said, if you are pregnant or simply concerned about the effects of these ingredients, do some research and look for safer options. There are more and more of them on the market.

WARNING: COMMON AND POSSIBLY HARMFUL INGREDIENTS

POSSIBLY CARCINOGENIC OR TOXIC INGREDIENTS	POTENTIALLY IRRITATING OR HARMFUL INGREDIENTS
Acrylates (acrylic-based thickeners)	Glycols (propylene, butylene, caprylyl, and hexylene)
Parabens (butylparaben, methylparaben, ethylparaben)	Silicones (dimethicone, cyclomethicone)
PEGS (polyethylene glycol—a petrochemical that can act as an emulsifier, a surfactant, or an emollient)	Alcohols (benzyl, ethyl, isopropyl)
Phthalates (synthetic polymers found in hair spray, fragrances, and nail polish)	Sulfites (sodium, potassium, ammonium)
Formaldehyde (found in nail polish)	Sodium laureth sulfate
Diazolidinyl and imidazolidinyl urea (a formaldehyde preservative)	Tetrasodium and disodium EDTA
Ethanolamines (diethanolamine, or DEA)	

The FDA does not require cosmetics to undergo approval before they are sold to the public. Only ingredients that are classified as drugs, elements that affect the structure or function of the body, are in any way regulated. These drugs are labeled as active ingredients above the cosmetic components, or inactive ingredients. The manufacturer must provide scientific proof to the FDA that active ingredients are safe and effective. As far as the cosmetic components go, they must be listed in descending order by quantity. So if water is the first ingredient listed, it's the most plentiful element in the product. If an antioxidant is last on the list, there's probably just a trace of it included. You should question whether that popular antioxidant or all-the-rage natural ingredient is mainly marketing or has been proven effective in the amount contained in the product. The question also arises how many of these ingredients, active or inactive, may actually penetrate to the dermis (and consequently be transported into the bloodstream). Can the paraben preservatives in all the lotions or creams we apply to our skin have some kind of negative effect if they do break through the skin's surface? Science hasn't yet been able to adequately answer that extremely important (and frightening) question. We should be as safety-conscious about what we put on our body as what we put inside it. The products we put on our skin are as important as the food we eat, and we should be aware of the untested, unregulated chemicals in both. So my best advice is to be aware of the ingredients in your products and be educated with the latest information available.

Web Sites for Reference

When you're in doubt about ingredients or specific skin care products, it's a good idea to check these informative sites to find some answers. They are great references to bookmark and visit frequently.

Environmental Working Group: www.ewg.org

www.cir-safety.org

The Campaign for Safe Cosmetics: www.safecosmetics.org

www.cosmeticsinfo.org

Skin Deep: www.cosmeticdatabase.com

Terralina (natural skin care products): www.terralina.com

www.ellenmarmur.com

>>> A REAL PATIENT STORY:
Are Baby Products Safer and Gentler?

A young woman recently came in with her four-month-old son. He was suffering from eczema, and in order to soothe his skin, she used an all-natural baby cream recommended for eczema and other skin sensitivities. Although it was labeled as hypoallergenic, noncomedogenic, and "for babies," it immediately caused her baby's skin to break out in a painful red rash. The main ingredients in the product—water, aloe vera, calendula, glycerin, vitamin E—were soothing and probably benign but the essential oils described as antibacterial might have been the irritant. The cream also has a strong smell, which is a good sign that it might not be as baby-friendly as you want it to be. (It also contains a trace amount of methylparaben preservative, which is potentially toxic in much larger amounts.) Essential oils can be extremely strong, especially on a baby's delicate skin. And extracts used for their antibacterial properties—eucalyptus, camphor, cinnamon, rosemary, and all citrus oils—are known to be potentially irritating. Because the baby product didn't list the specific oils or concentrations used (and didn't have to), there's no way of knowing which might have brought on the reaction. I recommended that she discontinue use of this particular product (which she had already done) and begin using either a topical steroid cream or a prescription anti-inflammatory such as tacrolimus or pimecrolimus. Theoretically, any skin care product made for babies should be safer and gentler, but there are no guarantees. Most of them contain similar ingredients as their adult counterparts, and they aren't necessarily better if they are natural or organic. It's always wise to read the label carefully (beware of essential oils, fragrances, and lots of chemical additives), and patch test the product first on your baby's belly.

Cosmetic Catchphrases

Let's begin with the big, bold print, the buzzwords right on the front label—terms such as "hypoallergenic" and "dermatologist-tested." What do they mean? Do they denote anything at all? These claims may sound technical and important, but they actually signify very little. (We've already learned that "100% Natural" doesn't necessarily mean what it states.) With no FDA standards to govern these definitions, and because manufacturers don't need to back up their claims, most of the time they guarantee nothing more than market value and a lot of hot air.

Hypoallergenic. The product is allegedly free of substances that are known to cause allergic reactions, so it should be less likely to cause irritation. Now that harsh ingredients are used less and less in most products, this term is becoming more meaningless. There is no scientific evidence to prove that hypoallergenic cosmetics are safer or produce less irritation.

PH balanced. The product is compatible with the neutral pH of the skin, so it won't react with it adversely. Some chemical ingredients, such as acids or alkaline detergents, change the pH balance temporarily and can affect the epidermal barrier. The phrase can be a decent guide to finding a gentle, basic skin care product that doesn't contain these elements.

Soap-free. The cleanser does not contain a highly alkaline detergent, but that doesn't mean it doesn't utilize a synthetic surfactant that may be drying or irritating to the skin. It's a good idea to check the ingredients list for one of the milder surfactants listed on pages 60–61.

Fragrance-free or unscented. This indicates that there are no chemical additives used specifically to create fragrance, but the product could still contain essential plant oils or extracts that mask the not-so-pretty smell of the core ingredients. So the product may actually have a scent (coming from the basic components), but nothing has been added for that purpose alone.

Noncomedogenic. The product is not supposed to contain anything that is known to block pores, namely, mineral oil, lanolin, paraffin or fatty acids. It may not be a fail-safe guarantee against breaking out, but it's a good term to look for if you have acne or oily skin.

Dermatologist-tested or -approved. A dermatologist tested the product in some way. One doctor, somewhere, used it (even if he or she didn't necessarily like it). It does not mean there was a clinical trial or that a group of dermatologists endorse it. As a dermatologist, I receive surveys all the time from well-known companies asking me which products I recommend. So when an advertisement states that "9 out of 10 dermatologists recommend" something, that's what it's based on.

Clinically proven or scientifically proven. "Clinically" means that testing of some kind was done on animals or people, while "scientifically" refers to testing in a laboratory. The manufacturers themselves usually do both, so you have to question the validity of the testing, since the data are not disclosed. You have to read the fine print—if it's there at all.

Oil-free. The product should contain no palm, coconut, olive, or plant oils, lanolin, or mineral oil. But it might include a thickening ingredient, such as isopropyl palmitate, that has a similar emollient effect (aka greasy feel) on the skin.

Translating the Ingredients List

Ingredients in a skin care product work in the same way as ingredients in a food recipe. For example, in baking, butter richens up a cookie recipe (believe it or not, avocado could even be used as a healthier fat substitute) in the same way that shea butter or fatty acids enrich a face cream. Cornstarch acts as a thickener and binder in cooking, just as an emulsifier such as stearic acid or cetyl alcohol in a cosmetic makes the texture smoother and holds oil and water together. All the various ingredients, whether in a cake or in a cleanser, must combine to create a harmonious whole.

The idea may be the same, but recipe ingredients are a lot easier to understand than the confusing chemical jargon on a product label (maybe because, with a recipe, we actually have to go out, buy the stuff, and put it all together in the kitchen ourselves). With big companies and chemists cooking up our skin care products, we need to be fairly well versed on what's included in the formula. Most product ingredients have a primary function, but quite often a single ingredient multitasks like crazy. For instance, cetyl and cetearyl alcohol are waxy, solid emollients that act as thickeners and emulsifiers in a product, and they moisturize the skin as a by-product. Stearic acid works as an emulsifier, but it's also a moisturizing and cleansing agent. Most ingredients not only benefit the skin in some way but also perform one or more big jobs that keep the product's delivery system intact.

What Ingredients Do

- They moisturize, using humectant and emollient ingredients.
- They bind, holding other ingredients together.
- They emulsify, blending oil and water substances together in a smooth formula.
- They thicken or smooth, making a formula richer or able to glide on more easily.
- They preserve, preventing the product from deteriorating, and harboring bacteria.
- They adjust the pH balance, acting as a buffer to stabilize acids and bases.

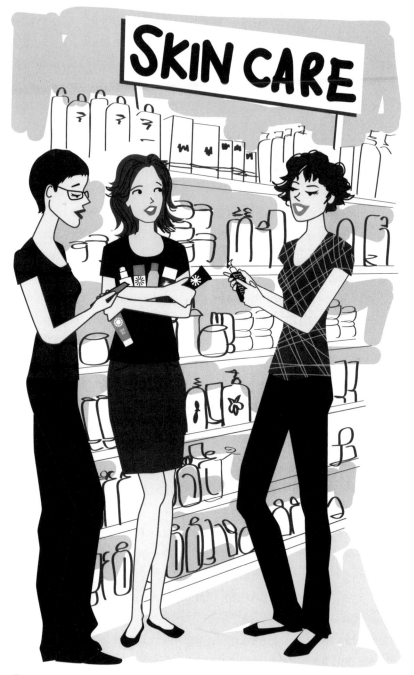

Start to read the back label on products. Look at the ingredients like you would a recipe. Find the active ingredients. Soon you will be able to do this for sunscreens and cosmeceuticals. Teach your friends!

Common Ingredients at a Glance:
A Primer on the Cosmetics Lexicon

Make some flash cards, memorize the ingredients, or just tear out this list. With it, you'll be able to look at any product label and know what each ingredient does in your cleanser or moisturizer and why it is there.

>>> EMOLLIENTS

Ingredients that soften skin and seal in moisture, creating an occlusive, protective barrier on the surface.

Shea butter

Cocoa butter

Mineral oil

Lanolin

Petrolatum

Paraffin

Beeswax

Squalene

Coconut, jojoba, sesame, almond, and other plant oils

Cetyl alcohol

Olive oil (oleic acid)

Triethylhexanoin

>>> HUMECTANTS:

Moisturizing ingredients that attract water to the skin.

Glycerin

Propylene glycol

Sorbitol

Sodium PCA

Hyaluronic acid

Allantoin (also acts as an anti-inflammatory agent)

Urea

>>> SURFACTANTS
"Surface active agents" that are used in cleansers to dissolve dirt and oils on the skin's surface; they also decrease the surface tension in a product, helping it to glide on easily.
Sodium laureth sulfate

Sodium cocyl isethionate

Cocomidopropyl betaine

Disodium cocamphodiacetate

Ammonium lauryl sulfate

Polysorbate 85 or polysorbate 60

Sodium lauryl sulfate

Cocamide DEA

>>> BINDERS AND EMULSIFIERS
Elements that create a stable mixture of different ingredients—binding oil and water together, for example:
Butylene glycol (also a humectant)

Polysorbates

Glyceryl stearate (also an emollient and adds pearlescence)

Cetearyl, cetyl, and stearyl alcohol (also a waxy emollient that adds opacity to color)

Stearic acid (also a surfactant and emollient and adds opacity to color)

PEG (polyethylene glycol for example, PEG-100 stearate) (also an emollient and surfactant)

Triethanolamine (also a buffer)

Palmitates (ethylhexyl, isopropyl, and cetyl palmitates are also emollients)

Ceteareth 20

>>> TEXTURIZERS
Substances that thicken or add slip to a product, so it can be applied smoothly. They literally add a rich texture to a cream or lotion.
Alkyl benzoate (also an emollient)

Carbomer

Polymers (in the form of either polyethylene glycol or natural polysaccharides such as seaweed)

Dimethicone, cyclomethicone (these silicones are also emollients)

Polysorbate 20 and 80 (also surfactants)

Pentaerythrityl tetraoctanoate

Caprylic and succinic triglycerides (also emollients)

Sodium chloride

>>> BUFFERS
Substances that neutralize acids, balance the pH of a product, and make it less irritating.
Sodium bicarbonate (baking soda)

Citric acid

Triethanolamine

>>> PRESERVATIVES
Ingredients that kill bacteria to prevent a product from contamination
Tocopherol acetate (vitamin E derivative; is also an emollient and antioxidant).

Propylene and butylene glycols (also humectants)

Disodium and tetrasodium EDTA

Diazolidinyl and imidazolydyl urea

Parabens (Methylparaben, polyparaben, butylparaben, etc.)

Phenoxyethanol

Methylisothiazolinone

Ascorbyl palmitate (a derivative of vitamin C)

Benzoic acid

Benzyl alcohol

Tear-out Cheat Sheets:
Ingredients to Look For, and Avoid, for Your Skin Tendency

IF YOUR SKIN IS GENERALLY OILY OR ACNE-PRONE

INGREDIENTS TO LOOK FOR	INGREDIENTS TO AVOID *WHY: THESE CAN CLOG PORES AND ADD OIL.*
> CLEANSER: Sodium laureth sulfate Sodium cocyl isethionate Cocomidopropyl betaine Disodium cocamphodiacetate > ACTIVE INGREDIENTS: Salicylic acid Benzoyl peroxide	*Emollients such as:* Shea butter Mineral oil Lanolin Petrolatum Paraffin Beeswax Squalene Oils Alkyl benzoate (an emollient thickener) Silcones Palmitates (ethylhexyl, isopropyl, and cetyl palmitates) Acrylate polymers (in sunscreens) Titanium dioxide Zinc oxide

IF YOUR SKIN IS GENERALLY DRY

INGREDIENTS TO LOOK FOR	**INGREDIENTS TO AVOID** ***WHY: THESE CAN BE DRYING OR TOO IRRITATING.***
> CLEANSER:	Isopropyl alcohol
Polysorbate 85 or 60	
Cocmidopropyl Betaine	Sodium chloride
> CLEANSER AND MOISTURIZER:	
Emollients such as:	*Surfactants such as:*
Shea or cocoa butter	Sodium lauryl sulfate
Lanolin	Sodium laureth sulfate
Petrolatum	Ammonium lauryl sulfate
Paraffin	
Beeswax	Soaps such as sodium tallowate or cocoate
Squalene	
Coconut, jojoba, sesame, almond, and other plant oils	Salicylic acid
Cetyl alcohol	Willow bark (the natural version of salicylic acid)
Olive oil (oleic acid)	
Triethylhexanoin	AHA acids
Humectants such as:	
Glycerin	
Propylene glycol	
Sorbitol	
Sodium PCA	
Hyaluronic acid	
Allantoin	
Urea	
> MOISTURIZING ADDITIVES (IN THE DELIVERY SYSTEM):	
Stearic acid	
Cetearyl alcohol	
Caprylic triglyceride	
Butylene glycol	

IF YOUR SKIN IS GENERALLY SENSITIVE

INGREDIENTS TO LOOK FOR	INGREDIENTS TO AVOID *WHY: THESE CAN BE HARSH OR IRRITATING.*
> CLEANSER: Polysorbate 85 or 60	Isopropyl alcohol
> MOISTURIZER: *Emollients (to protect) such as:* Shea or cocoa butter Lanolin Petrolatum Paraffin Beeswax Squalene Coconut, jojoba, sesame, almond, and other plant oils Cetyl alcohol Olive oil (oleic acid) Triethylhexanoin	Sodium chloride *Surfactants such as:* Sodium lauryl sulfate Sodium laureth sulfate Ammonium lauryl sulfate *Soaps such as sodium tallowate or cocoate* Salicylic acid Willow bark (the natural version of salicylic acid)
Humectants such as: Glycerin Propylene glycol Sorbitol Sodium PCA Hyaluronic acid Allantoin Urea	AHA acids *Chemical sunscreens such as:* Avobenzone Octinoxate Octisalate Homosalate Octocrylene Oxybenzone
Anti-inflammatory additives: Tocopherol acetate Chamomile and cucumber extracts	

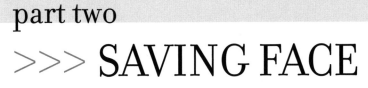

part two

>>> SAVING FACE

The Health of Your Skin

5

Your UV Protection Strategy: On the Beach, at the Pool, in the Sun Anywhere

The sun is not a bad, scary thing. It feels wonderful, addictively so (as you learned in the last chapter), and a sunny day makes everyone want to go outside to enjoy it. No one wants to think about his or her body being under attack from the sun—even though it is. But there are so many effective tools to protect us that we don't have to give up that euphoric feeling we get in the sunshine. Not putting your skin at risk is simply a matter of using sunscreen and some common sense.

If sun protection products don't work successfully, the fault is really our own. Most of us aren't using them (1) correctly, (2) in adequate amounts, or (3) at all. Studies have shown that most people put on only a fraction of the sunscreen they should, which is one of the main reasons it fails to deliver the SPF we expect. *Consumer Reports* states that people typically apply about 25 to 75 percent less sunscreen than the amount used in product testing, so if you apply an SPF 30 sparingly (who wants to feel greasy or have an opaque film on the skin?), you're probably getting closer to an SPF 10. A 2005 study assessed the level of sunscreen use in male college athletes. During one week, 85 percent reported using no sunscreen at all, and only 6 percent used sunscreen but only for three out of the seven days.[1] To get the labeled SPF protection, an adult needs to use a shot glass full of sunscreen all over, or one teaspoon of product over each body part (each thigh, shin, each arm, back, front chest, and torso, neck, face).

Remember that sunscreen is used up over time. So one application before you go to the beach shouldn't be the last time you put it on. It must be reapplied every one to two hours. It doesn't matter if the label states that the product is "water-resistant" or "sweatproof." Every time you go in the water, reapply it afterward. As sticky as that sunscreen may feel on your skin, it's not glued onto your body, and a good portion of it can rub off, sweat off, or rinse off. Also, just because you use a higher SPF, it doesn't mean it's okay to bake yourself longer. The goal of sunscreen shouldn't be to prolong the amount of time you can fry yourself in the sun, and no sunscreen can completely prevent all possible damage from ultraviolet rays. Yet we all seem to be in denial about sunscreen math. A 1999 study published in the *Journal of the National Cancer Institute* showed that using higher-SPF sunscreens led to increased sun exposure. In the experiment, one group was given a low-SPF sunscreen, while the other used SPF 30. The group given the higher SPF spent 20 percent more time in the sun than the other group.[2] Even though it's wrong-headed, we're often guilty of spending more time in the sun than we should and not reapplying a sunscreen just because the SPF is 50 or 70. Those are deceptive numbers for sure, and inaccurate—especially if you remember that a higher SPF gives you only a fraction more protection. In fact, for these reasons, the FDA is considering limiting SPF values to 30, with higher SPFs labeled "30 plus."

>>> **A REAL PATIENT STORY:**
Beach Culture—Denial Runs in Families

I take care of a lot of doctors and their families. One of my patients is a tall, dark, and handsome doctor (emphasis on the "dark"). Because he's deeply tan all year round, I couldn't help but give him my lecture when he came in for his annual skin check. (When I see someone with a bronze tan, I find it distressing, like examining someone with a wheezing cough. As a physician, I recognize it as a sign of a possible health problem, and I want to help.) This doctor and his family spend all summer at their beach house and long days in the sun. I told him, "You don't realize it now, you're young and everything is perfect, but you are getting way too much sun." He gave me a guilty smile, told me that he wears sunscreen, knows about the dangers of sun damage, but had no intention of changing his beach lifestyle. "The kids love to spend the day on the beach. It's our family time, it's what we love to do together." This is a person at the highest level of medical education, and he was in absolute denial. The truth is, even if you re-apply sunscreen, you are getting too much UV radiation if you spend every day, all day, intentionally in the sun. This extreme puts your entire family in danger.

When this man's wife came in for a skin check, I gave her the same lecture and got the same response. On her body I found a possible melanoma that needed to be biopsied. She had a terrible, scared look on her face and asked, "How did this happen?" As if she had never heard all those lectures and all that knowledge. She ended up having a severely dysplastic nevus, a premelanoma, that was surgically excised. Right away, after this big reality check, she sent her kids in to be examined. Their friends started coming in to get their skin looked at too. (One ended up having several basal cell carcinomas that I had to remove.) This is a family for which not only changing their habits but altering their entire lifestyle mattered. It takes just one person in a family to speak some sense to everybody else and, in this case, also spread the word about a safer philosophy to friends. This one family successfully changed, and you can too.

We can all be sun optimists at times—armed with a million excuses for not wearing or reapplying sunscreen. Here's my top ten.

Top Ten List: You Know You're a Sun Optimist
if You Believe One of These Myths

1. You don't need sunscreen on a rainy or cloudy day.

2. A tan is fine, as long as you don't burn.

3. You're safe in the shade and don't need to wear sunscreen.

4. You don't need sunscreen on a plane, in a car, or in the house.

5. You need a serious sunscreen only if you're lying out at the beach or by the pool, not when you're on a walk or a bike ride.

- Moving around does not diminish sun damage. UV rays follow you no matter how fast you run. Always wear broad-spectrum sun protection when you walk, run, play tennis, golf, surf, or enjoy any outdoor activity at all.

6. A tan or naturally dark skin guards your skin from sun damage because of melanin production.

7. The faux tan you get from self-tanner also protects your skin because of the production of melanin.

- The chemical dihydroxyacetone, or DHA, interacts with skin cells on the skin's surface to change their color. It has nothing to do with melanin production. The fact is, unless a self-tanner has added sun protection in it (and some do), it won't shield your skin at all. (Be aware that sunless tanner tends to collect and concentrate in the pores, and the DHA can make them appear dirty, even though it doesn't actually cause blackheads or acne.)

8. Tanning booths are safer than baking in the sun outside.

- It's proven that people who use artificial sun lamps or tanning booths are 2.5 times more likely to develop squamous cell carcinoma, 1.5 times more likely to get basal cell carcinoma, and at much higher risk for melanoma than those who do not use them.[3] The American Academy of Dermatology launched a public service advertising campaign with the theme "Indoor Tanning Is Out." Hopefully it will encourage indoor tanners, especially the girls and young women aged sixteen to twenty-nine who make up the 70 percent majority, to think twice.

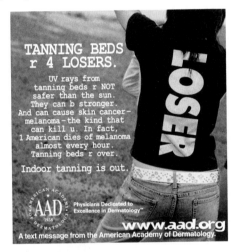

9. Since 80 percent of your sun exposure happens before you're eighteen, it's too late to bother with sunscreen now.

- That percentage is now known to be incorrect. I don't know where this statistic came from in the first place. Anyway, it is no excuse not to protect your skin right now.

10. Wearing a higher SPF (above 30) will protect your skin twice as long and twice as effectively.

Which of these statements is true? Not one.

How to Apply Sunscreen

The best technique for an even application of sunscreen is to dab it on
in little dots all over one area (such as your face, neck, and ears). Once
your dots are in place, rub them in and move on to the next area. This
way you can see exactly where you've applied the lotion, so you don't
miss any spots. Apply it mindfully and thoroughly from head to toe, or
vice versa, so you don't forget any areas. If you skip around, it's too
easy to forget where you've applied or not, in case you're interrupted
(the phone rings, one of your kids needs you, the toast is burning,
anything!).

Do you have to apply sunscreen at least thirty minutes before
going into the sun, so it has a chance to absorb into your skin? I
think that's a myth (since sunscreens, especially physical blocks such
as titanium dioxide and zinc, are effective right away), but it's vital to
apply it before you go outside. The five minutes you spend walking
to the pool, the beach, the tennis court are five minutes your skin is
left totally unprotected. The best thing to do is put on sunscreen
when you're naked. Put those dots everywhere and blend them in
before you put on your swimsuit or clothes. Clothing tends to shift
and move as you do—whether a bathing suit, tank top, shorts, or
sundress—so you want to protect every inch of skin (even underneath your clothing, which has only an SPF of 2 or 5) if you're in
direct sun, just in case.

We are getting used to applying sunscreen on most exposed body
parts, such as the face, arms, chest, and legs. But do you remember
your hairline, ears (and inside them), scalp (if you've ever had a sunburn there you won't forget again), and hands and feet? Believe me,
I've taken off plenty of skin cancers from the soles of the feet, between
the toes, on the ankles. Every day at work I operate on skin cancers
that are located on neglected areas of the skin. Five or six hundred of
my seven hundred annual Mohs skin cancer surgeries are on parts of
the body where sunscreen should be applied but isn't: eyelids, inside

the ears, lips. Melanoma also affects nails, so you want to protect your fingernails and toenails and cuticles too. Here's a checklist of hard-to-remember spots. Make sure you cover these areas, on yourself and your family.

Spots Not to Skip

✓ The scalp (your hairline or part)—wearing a hat works best!
✓ Ears (lobes, inside the ears)
✓ Neck
✓ Hands (palms, in between fingers, nails)
✓ Feet (soles, in between toes, on nails)
✓ Lips
✓ Around the eyes
✓ Insides of the arms

New Sunscreen Labeling May Be on the Horizon

With the recent knowledge of the dangers of UVA rays, the old SPF rating system seems inadequate, giving us only half the information we need (namely about UVB protection only). The FDA plans to institute a new and improved system that measures UVA protection too. It proposes to show the SPF number along with a four-star UVA rating on sunscreen labels—one star being low protection and four meaning the highest UVA protection. (If the product does not have any UVA protection, it must state "No UVA Protection" on the label.) It would also prohibit use of the terms "waterproof" and "sunblock" on a label, as they mislead consumers into thinking a product won't come off in water or will block all UV rays. Because sunscreen manufacturers are contesting these proposed rules, the FDA has not set a date to make the updated regulations final or to implement them.

Sun Protection Add-ons: These Are Not Optional

Sunscreen is only part of the story. We need to use other tools to help protect ourselves in the sun. Sitting under an umbrella, avoiding the strongest midday sun, and wearing a broad-brimmed hat (6-inch minimum) all add to your sun protection factor. Here are three other smart solutions that go even further to help safeguard your lips, your eyes, and your whole body.

Broad-Spectrum Lip Balm

At least once a week I remove a skin cancer from someone's upper lip. Because the skin on the lips is thinner, it is more vulnerable than the rest of your body. Also, because lips have no melanin, they are left unshielded. (It's the blood vessels just beneath the surface of the lips that provide their rosy color). We know that sun exposure destroys collagen, so it thins the lips over time. Wearing an SPF lip balm every day protects the skin and the collagen beneath it, in exactly the same way that regular sunscreen use prevents future sagging and aging of the skin on your face and body.

A recent study found that less than 25 percent of Americans use some form of lip protection. (But I don't know one man, except my husband, who applies a lip balm with SPF, do you?) When you're in direct sun—whether on the beach, driving in a convertible, or sitting outside at a baseball game—wear a lip balm with a broad-spectrum sunscreen. Lipstick or gloss is not a sun shield just because it's layered on top of the lips. Indeed, it can make matters much worse. The same study that reported the low percentage of people protecting their lips, done at Baylor University Medical Center in Dallas, also found that shiny lip gloss attracts light (and ultraviolet radiation) and increases a person's risk of skin cancer. Many glosses and lipsticks contain an SPF. However, these cosmetics often include only a UVB filter such as octinoxate and no UVA protection at all. As always, read the label carefully.

UV-Protective Sunglasses

Sunglasses = sunblock. Not only can a pair of shades look cool (the bigger and darker, the better!), but lenses that have "98–100% UV protection" help prevent skin cancer. If the sunglasses don't carry the American Optometric Association's Seal of Acceptance, have them tested at the store with a photometer that measures the lenses' UV protection. If the shades you like don't offer at least 98 percent protection, you can ask your optometrist to add a UV coating to the lenses.

The delicate skin of the eyelids and around the eyes is extremely vulnerable. Basal and squamous cell carcinomas are common on eyelids, and about 2 percent of all skin cancers including melanoma, are in the eye. Sun damage also increases the risk of cataracts, macular degeneration, and retinal injury. On a more superficial front, all that squinting in the sun adds up to crow's feet and furrows between the brows later on. Understandably, many people don't like to wear sunscreen close to their eyes because it stings (although formulations made especially for babies and those with sensitive skin may be worth a try). In lieu of that, it's even more mandatory to wear sunglasses every day since they provide a perfect physical block against UV rays. Big, wrap-around types aren't just stylish; they shield more of your face.

Sun-Protective Clothing

Like sunglasses, the right kind of clothing provides an effective physical block to the sun. But a white T-shirt won't do much good; it has an SPF of only 5 (and when wet it goes down to SPF 2). Darker colors absorb more light, and tighter-constructed fabrics are better barriers. I think UV-protective clothing is just as important as sunscreen, and it's an easy way to make sure that you and your kids are protected when you're outside. (It's also a smart idea to wear a sun-protective swimsuit.) Sun-protective fabric is engineered specifically to block and absorb ultraviolet light. It has a tight, nonporous weave (usually light-weight polyester, nylon, cotton jersey, or linen), and the material is infused with sunscreens (such as titanium dioxide and zinc microfibers).

The Federal Trade Commission (FTC) and the Consumer Products Safety Commission (CPSC) are involved in regulating UV-protective wear, and the FDA regulates these fabrics in much the same way as it does sunscreen products (since they contain a "medical active ingredient"). Sun-protective clothing should carry a "UPF" (ultraviolet protection factor) rating. Unlike the SPF on sunscreen products, this measures the protection provided from both UVA *and* UVB. Most sun-protective clothing has a UPF of 30+ to 50+ (the maximum level blocks 98 percent of UV radiation). These fabrics are also durability-tested, so the protection can't wear off or be washed out of the clothing, even if you launder it a hundred times.

Another option is to wash your regular clothes with SunGuard, a laundry additive that treats fabric with the sunscreen Tinosorb. When added to detergent, it provides the clothing being washed with approximately 96 percent UPF protection (bumping that white T-shirt's UPF from 5 up to 30). The treated clothes will retain that UPF level through about twenty washings.

Three sun-protective clothing companies to check out are:
Coolibar: www.coolibar.com

Solumbra: www.solumbra.com

SunGuard: www.sunguardsunprotection.com

How Sun Damages the Skin

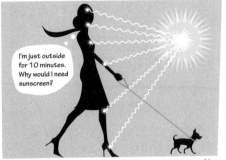

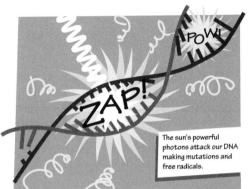

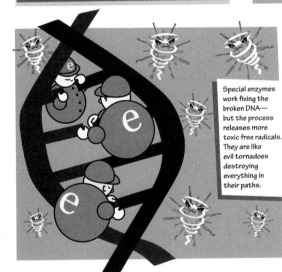

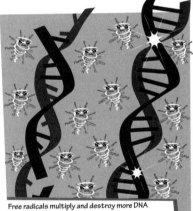

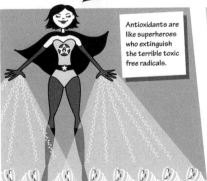

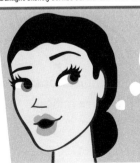

>>> q&a

Q: How does sun damage the DNA in the first place? And what are free radicals? Are they just a marketing term?

A: Free radicals may sound like some kind of rock band, but they are toxic by-products in the body. To make a very long and complex scientific phenomenon short, this is how they are produced through UV damage to a cell's DNA.

A photon (the sun's laser beam) zaps through the cell membrane and the cytoplasm, through the nuclear membrane (the safe, womb-like center of the cell), and hits the DNA. Imagine DNA as being like two pieces of spaghetti laid parallel, with crosshatches all the way along like a ladder, then rolled up and twisted like an intricately knotted cuff link. When a photon burns a hole into the DNA knot, it starts to unravel and the two sides of the ladder begin opening up. The immune system immediately sends out enzymes to fix the problem. (Enzymes are proteins that act as workers in the body, fixing damage by causing chemical reactions.) One enzyme comes in and gobbles up the damaged portion; then it creates a new DNA rung to fix that ladder. Another enzyme double-checks it, another seals it all together, and another wraps it up into a nice, perfect knot again. All these chemical reactions done to reconstruct damaged DNA give off toxic oxygen by-products, or free radicals. Oxygen can be stable, with two electrons in its orbit, or, if it has only one electron (as free radicals do), it's on fire—trying to steal an electron from another molecule in order to become stable. An unstable oxygen molecule races around like a toddler with a pair of scissors or a Tasmanian devil, causing destruction to anything in its path until it runs out of energy. Antioxidants quench and destroy that toxic free radical.

Antioxidants: The Big Boost

Antioxidants in certain foods—green tea, olive oil, blueberries, salmon or sunflower seeds—act like superhero nutrients in the body. They extinguish toxic oxygen molecules known as free radicals, the bad by-products of cell renewal that are also produced by pollution and sun damage.

Antioxidants may turn out to be even more powerful defenders than we thought, and researchers are studying their potential as cancer fighters and UV protectors. Scientific studies seem to come out every day, touting the near-miraculous sun-protective and cancer-preventive benefits of antioxidant compounds in everything from pomegranates to red wine. The polyphenols in green tea have been proven to protect the DNA in skin cells in mice from UV damage, to protect skin against sunburns, and possibly to help prevent basal and squamous cell carcinomas. In a National Cancer Institute study done at the University of Illinois, the antioxidant compound resveratrol (found in cranberries, red wine, and grapes) inhibited the development of cancers in mice. (The antioxidant's beneficial effects on humans are still uncertain.) Antioxidant compounds found in pomegranates have also shown a great ability to inhibit tumor production and growth. A study published in *The Journal of Investigative Dermatology* found that vitamin C and E supplements taken for three months significantly reduced sunburns and sun damage.[4] Here's the latest news presented at the British Society for Investigative Dermatology. A team of British researchers found that eating tomato paste and olive oil protected skin against UV radiation. In this human study, the volunteers who ate a spaghetti sauce of cooked tomatoes and olive oil every day for three months had 33 percent more protection against sunburn than the participants who were given only olive oil on their pasta. It's believed that the antioxidant compound lycopene, found in high concentration in cooked tomatoes, is the reason for the apparent skin benefit.

Researchers are constantly searching for new and novel ways to battle disease and safeguard our bodies from harmful elements (such as ultraviolet radiation), but we need to understand that most of this research is still far from finished. The majority has been done via lab or animal studies, so the effects of topical or ingested antioxidants on the human body are still quite inconclusive. My advice: eat a balanced, healthy diet with lots of fresh fruits and vegetables, drink green tea instead of soda, have a glass of red wine rather than another cocktail, and why not have tomato sauce on your ravioli? But don't make yourself crazy, and don't overdo it with supplements. Taking too much of any vitamin or antioxidant pill can be toxic because the body can store up an overdose of chemical compounds—a medical condition called "hypervitaminosis" or vitamin poisoning. Believe me, I've been there. I know firsthand that overdoing a good thing, such as antioxidants, can go wrong. I went overboard eating salmon for one week—for breakfast, lunch, and dinner—partially because I bought into the hype about salmon as a superfood, high in antioxidants and omega-3 fatty acids. And it is a highly healthy fish to eat—in moderation. By the third day of my salmon binge, I had extreme pain in my left big toe, to the point where it woke me up at night. My toe was red and throbbing and hurt so much that the weight of a sheet on top of it was excruciating. I was diagnosed with gout. Yes, gout, the disease of gluttony that I assumed afflicted only portly men in generations past. Gout is due to the buildup and crystallization of uric acid (a natural antioxidant) in the joint. Uric acid is metabolized in the body from purines (found in high concentrations in salmon). My elevated uric acid level actually gave me gout! When I stopped eating so much salmon, the swelling and pain in my toe went away.

Many animal and lab studies have concentrated on the topical use of antioxidants. Can green tea, vitamin C or E, pomegranate, or red wine have the same positive effects on the skin when applied on top of it? The jury is definitely still out, although every cosmetic company promotes the inclusion of antioxidant ingredients in its products. Widely used, common antioxidant derivatives such as ascorbic acid and tocopherol acetate are advertised as vitamin C and vitamin E antioxidants. But which antioxidants, if any, are included in high enough concentrations to truly be effective when used topically? Are they stable enough to remain active when they oxidize in the open air and are put on the skin? And can topical antioxidants actually penetrate to the dermis to have an effect on the DNA of skin cells? I think these nutrients are far more stable and effective when they are ingested as food in your diet. That way they are delivered to the dermis through the circulatory system. I trust my internal systems more than chemists who are putting antioxidants (in questionable amounts and questionably stable forms) into lotions and creams. The body is efficient about how it breaks down and delivers nutrients to our skin—it's a more reliable messenger.

All that said, eating a diet rich in antioxidants, using a moisturizer that contains them, and drinking green tea aren't bad ideas—and they might make a difference in boosting your protection from sun damage and possibly skin cancer. Antioxidants are so popular—indeed, ubiquitous—in the current beauty market that new antioxidant labeling is beginning to appear on skin care products. An EPF (environmental protection factor) rating measures an antioxidant's potency and effectiveness on a scale of 1 to 100 (100 being the strongest and most powerful against sun, pollution, and free-radical damage). The rating is based on a 2005 study that compared topical antioxidants by their ability to protect the skin.[5] (The antioxidant idebenone scored 95, vitamin E 80, and Vitamin C 52.) This study laid out the scientific methods used to quantify the rankings, but new evaluations will have to be done to test newer antioxidants (such as green tea, pomegranate, and CoffeeBerry) that were not involved in the original study.

Another interesting antioxidant option that's garnering a lot of excitement is a nonprescription dietary supplement called Heliocare.

Bear with me because this one sounds even wackier than daily doses of pasta sauce—but there may be something to it. The pills contain an extract from a South American tropical fern (*Polypodium leucotomos*), which has been found to ward off sunburn if taken regularly. A 2004 study done by Harvard University scientists discovered that the pills dramatically decreased redness in the skin of human subjects.[6] Another clinical test found that after oral administration of *Polypodium leucotomos*, there was increased photoprotection of immune (Langerhans) cells.[7] The science behind this new antioxidant supplement is pretty solid, and, if taken correctly, it could help prevent sun damage. I have patients who take Heliocare, and they do notice less sunburn.

The only bad thing about all of this is that people might think they can simply take a pill rather than putting on sunscreen. All these wonderful antioxidant boosters should *not* be used in lieu of being sun smart (i.e., wearing sunscreen). They are meant to up the ante of your sun protection, not replace it. Please do not think you can slack off on sunscreen, bask in the sun, and undo the damage by popping a vitamin E capsule, drinking some green tea, or applying an antioxidant lotion. Even if antioxidants can help enhance sun protection and decrease sun damage, they shouldn't be considered some kind of morning-after antidote to an irresponsible day at the beach.

Adding controversy and confusion to the optimistic antioxidant story is a 2007 French study published in *The Journal of Nutrition* that found that taking an antioxidant supplement including vitamins C and E could increase women's risk of skin cancer by 68 percent.[8] And the risk of melanoma was four times greater for women taking these supplements. The scientists involved 13,000 men and women between the ages of thirty-five and sixty. Half took an oral antioxidant supplement once a day, and the other half took a placebo. After more than seven years, fifty-one women taking antioxidant supplements developed skin cancer, while thirty in the placebo group did. Among the men, thirty-three in the antioxidant group got skin cancer and forty-three placebo takers did not. Perhaps the antioxidant-taking group failed to protect themselves with sunscreen (the study did not take sunscreen use into account), maybe they (mistakenly) believed that antioxidants were enough protection, or maybe they simply suffered more sun damage or bad genetic luck than the placebo group. Certainly the antioxidants were given to older individuals who had already suffered years of sun exposure. This study suggests that antioxidants aren't beneficial against sun protection and calls the taking of supplements into question, but it doesn't imply that antioxidants instigated skin cancer. Personally, I feel that eating a diet rich in antioxidants is beneficial for the body and may help fight free radical damage from sun exposure. But relying on antioxidant supplements or creams to counteract damage that's already been done (and not protecting your skin with sunscreen because of them) is an absurd—and extremely dangerous—gamble.

>>> skin lie: If you wear sunscreen, you won't get enough vitamin D.

>>> skin truth: Making vitamin D is one of the skin's big jobs, and it is certainly important for the absorption of calcium that builds strong bones. The vitamin also has beneficial effects on the body's immune system. In order to synthesize vitamin D through the skin, you do need some sun every day— but that doesn't mean you should bask in it unprotected. Five to fifteen minutes of incidental light is enough to get your body to make vitamin D. With the amount of sunscreen that you wear daily—be honest, probably a sheer coat of SPF 15 moisturizer—you will still get enough UV radiation to convert vitamin D in the skin. Remember, we still get the vitamin from milk and vitamin D–fortified foods like orange juice, milk, and cereals. Realistically, even if you

wear a moisturizer with SPF protection, you'll probably make enough vitamin D as you walk to the store or to work. Unless you slather on sunscreen like cake frosting from head to toe, sufficient UV rays will still penetrate your skin even with sunscreen on. It has been proven that normal vitamin D production levels can be maintained despite rigorous photoprotection.[9] It's important to note that photosynthesis of the vitamin can happen anywhere on the body, such as in your scalp or your hands. The worry about vitamin D deficiency is most relevant to people who are unable to go outside much. For most of us, it's not as significant a concern as UV radiation is.

>>>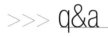

Q: Is it dangerous to put sunscreen on my infant?

A: I too have always read and believed that you shouldn't apply sunscreen to an infant's skin before the age of six months. The worry was that a baby's skin will absorb and react to harsh chemical ingredients more readily than an older child's. Now I don't necessarily agree with that thinking. Here's what I recommend (as a dermatologist and a mom): I would use a sunscreen on my baby if he or she were outside in direct sunlight. I'd make sure to use a mineral sunblock such as zinc oxide or titanium dioxide that is gentler on the skin. But try to avoid micronized or nanosized ingredients. And the formulation should be baby-safe, with more natural than synthetic ingredients. Even better, make sure your infant avoids the direct sun completely. But if you're going to be outside for an extended period of time with your child, you must protect his or her skin. Make sure your baby wears a hat and stays under an umbrella or a sun-protective tent. Remember, your child is still getting sun even in the shade, and a covered baby stroller offers no more protection than an umbrella.

One of the many responsibilities of being a parent is making sure your kids are protected in the sun. As they get a little bit older and spend more of their playtime outdoors, they desperately need you to apply sunscreen to their skin every day—and make them wear sun-protective clothes too. My kids actually *ask* for sunscreen when it's sunny. In intense sun, they feel more comfortable when they have on sun protection lotion. It's not brainwashing, I promise! Here's my secret: I use Banana Boat Kids Quik Blok Sunblock Spray Lotion and let my children spray paint on each other's skin and then rub it in. This trick delights them—it works like a charm.

Skin cancer is a disease generated by lots of cumulative sun damage (starting in childhood), and it doesn't just happen to grown-ups either. I've done my share of skin cancer surgeries on kids under the age of ten. Pediatric melanoma is still relatively uncommon, but it is alarmingly on the rise. Also, it is believed that DNA damage to skin cells less than thirty-five years old increases skin cancer risk later. Make sure your child is safe in the sun from birth on up.

Q: What if the worst-case scenario happens and I do get a sunburn? How should I take care of it?

A: Sunburn is a massive trauma to the skin, a major 911. When you really understand what a sunburn is, I promise you will do everything you can to prevent it from happening again. The reason your skin is hot is that the sun is not only cooking you from the outside but also causing your blood vessels to dilate fully. That redness is 100 percent due to increased vasodilation, rushing all of your repair mechanisms to the skin through the circulatory system. When you blister, it's because there's a shift of fluid from where it should be, in the cells and blood vessels, to the skin tissue, making it bubble up. A sunburn also kills basal cells, which then lose their ability to grip on to the dermis, and the loosening of the epidermis from the dermis generates blisters too. Have I scared you yet? Good. This is a very real, and very dangerous, injury. To make matters worse, sunburn continues to develop for twelve to twenty-four hours *after* the initial burn takes place. It's no wonder that a sunburn (or a lot of them) can lead to skin cancer.

A burn is a huge inflammatory response by the body; so if you do get one, take two aspirins to lessen the inflammation. The best topical antidote is fresh aloe vera, since it has anti-inflammatory and humectant properties. (Be careful of aloe vera gels or creams, as they may contain alcohol, which is dehydrating, and stick with pure aloe instead.) Along with alcohol, avoid products containing witch hazel, menthol, peppermint, and calamine lotion. And disregard the old wives' tale of putting milk on a sunburn—the lactic acid will exfoliate the injured epidermis. You want to use soothing creams with emollients such as shea butter or olive oil and anti-inflammatory ingredients such as cucumber, aloe, and allantoin. Hydrocortisone cream can be very helpful, but the 1 percent over-the-counter strength is probably not going to do it for you. You may need a doctor's prescription for a stronger concentration. Cold compresses will cool you down, but make sure they are moisturized with aloe or a rich cream. Plain water feels good initially, but when it evaporates, it dehydrates the skin and makes it feel even worse than before.

Q: Are there medications or topical treatments that will make my skin more likely to burn during my summer vacation?

A: Many medications can cause photosensitivity in some people. The photoreaction can mimic a sunburn or bring on an allergic reaction such as hives or a rash. Be sure to check with your pharmacist or doctor about what sun-related side effects your medications could give you. Antibiotics such as tetracycline and sulfamethoxazole (Bactrim), some diuretics and antihistamines (such as Benadryl), nonsteroidal anti-inflammatory drugs (Feldene, Naproxen, Motrin), and some antidepressants can be phototoxic after exposure to UV light. Researchers have found that taking these drugs also increases the risk of skin cancer if you are exposed to the sun.

It's easier to control the use of topical products because they are not essential to maintaining your health. Retinoids such as Retin-A, any AHA, even facial scrubs—anything that exfoliates the top layer of your skin—will make you more vulnerable to the elements. You should probably stop using any of them one week before going on a beach vacation. If the stratum corneum doesn't have that dead keratinocyte barrier on top of it, you're setting the skin up for irritation by salt water, chlorine, wind, and most of all the sun.

6

What Does a Dermatologist Do?
How Can I Be a Wiser Patient?
And Other Important Questions

I am often asked what a dermatologist does, why you need to see one regularly, and how you can choose the right one, among so many other questions. This is my opportunity to answer those questions.

The most important piece of advice I can give you, from a medical perspective, is to see a dermatologist once a year for a skin exam. Have your children checked annually from infancy on up too. It is the best way to spot skin cancers early, and if they *are* caught early, skin cancers are 100 percent curable. It takes just a few minutes once a year to gain peace of mind about your skin. In fact, a study published in the *Archives of Dermatology* reported that a full-body skin exam can be completed effectively in less than three minutes. Three minutes once a year is easy, it's doable, it's not a huge investment, and the American Academy of Dermatology even offers free screenings across the United States. (Go to www.aad.org for more information.) There's no excuse not to.

>>> q&a

Q: What does a dermatologist do?

A: Dermatology is a medical and surgical field specializing in the treatment of skin, hair, and nails and how they relate to your body as a whole. I diagnose and treat specific conditions of the skin and also use the skin as a map to see what's happening inside the body. I specialize in skin cancer, so I do a lot of skin checks concerning moles and red spots. And I do surgery to remove those if they are malignant. I also focus on cosmetic procedures such as laser surgery and injectable fillers and Botox. I feel that a huge part of what I do is educating patients. This way I can help my patients become participants in their own skin care. I prepare handouts in response to the questions that come up repeatedly: What's the difference between sunblock and sunscreen? How should I do a self-skin check? Another information sheet is all about skin cancer basics. And for every procedure that I do, I have a little pamphlet explaining what it is, what the side effects may be, its risks, and its benefits.

Q: How can I find a good dermatologist? Is it based on what hospital he or she is associated with or where he or she went to medical school?

A: I think both of those things are important. You want to look for a board-certified dermatologist. This means he or she has completed medical school, a three-year residency in dermatology and passed a rigorous two-part exam administered by the American Board of Dermatology, and are retested every ten years. Dermatology is one of the hardest and most competitive medical fields to get into. *The New York Times* recently reported that medical students accepted into dermatology residencies had the highest median medical board scores and the highest percentage of members in the medical honor society of eighteen specialties. So you are sure to find a wonderful physician if you do just a little bit of homework. Check the American Academy of Dermatology Web site (www.aad.org): its doctor locator function can supply a great list of board-certified dermatologists in your area. It's an excellent resource for information on physicians, skin conditions, and the latest research in the field of dermatology.

One factor that should probably not figure into your decision is the popular press. You shouldn't count out a doctor simply because he or she is not well known. In fact, some of the most brilliant dermatologists shy away from publicity or stay within the walls of academia. I think it's far more important to find somebody accessible who can spend an adequate amount of time with you and who will answer your questions thoughtfully. Ideally, you want a doctor you can feel comfortable with, someone resourceful enough to find answers for you if he or she doesn't know them and who can give you and your family good advice in the future. How you get along with your physician is key. After all, this is a relationship based on communication.

Q: What other questions should I ask the dermatologist?

A: You can ask what procedures the dermatologist specializes in. How often does he or she perform laser treatments or peels, liposuction, or other cosmetic procedures such as Botox or injectable fillers? Does the physician usually perform these procedures personally or have dermatologically trained registered nurses or residents do them? (In chapter 10, "The Big Breakthroughs," I will provide a comprehensive checklist of important questions to ask your doctor or the office staff before you go in for laser treatments, injectables, or a chemical peel.)

Don't be shy about asking a doctor about his or her credentials. (Most of us are happy to tell you about them.) You can do some sleuthing online to acquire information about a doctor's background. Find out what the dermatologist specializes in. Is it skin cancer surgery, cosmetic dermatology, or both? Is he or she affiliated with a hospital or medical group? Where did he or she train in residency? Did this physician do any subsequent fellowships or study under another doctor as a mentor? Has he or she published research papers, and where? Does the dermatologist teach or lecture regularly?

Q: When should I see a dermatologist for the first time? And why go if I don't have a skin problem?

A: The primary reason to go to a dermatologist, unless you have a medical issue, is to get a clean bill of health skin cancer-wise. A total body exam is mandatory once a year, every year—starting at age zero. If you have a one-year-old, take your baby to get an annual dermatologic checkup by a dermatologist. It's not fair to put that responsibility on a pediatrician. Because they weren't trained as extensively in dermatology, most don't do thorough skin exams (nor should they). I educate parents about what to look for on their children's skin—which brown spots are perfectly normal and how to tell if something might be suspicious. Also, eczema is usually worse in the first ten years of life. There are good treatments for it and great home therapies that a dermatologist can tell you about. Birthmarks, such as port wine stains, can be corrected with laser treatments much more easily and effectively at a younger age. In a nutshell, the earlier you start treatment and checkups, the better.

Most people don't get regular skin checks, and most don't take dermatological checkups as seriously as their yearly trip to the gynecologist or the dentist, even though they are equally important to your overall health. In 2004, the American Cancer Society found that just 20 percent of women surveyed had annual skin cancer screenings. That percentage was lower than the rate of participation in annual screenings for other types of cancer, such as yearly mammography for breast cancer. Another study, published in the *Journal of the American Academy of Dermatology*, found that only 15 percent of U.S. outdoor workers (those in construction, fishing, farming, and forestry) ever had a skin examination during their lifetimes. Not only do people in high-risk sun exposure occupations fail to get screened, but so do people who should know better. I have one patient, a successful beauty editor and writer, who had never gone to a dermatologist's office in her life before the age of thirty-six. This is a woman who writes about skin care for a living!

Few people see a dermatologist regularly unless they have acne or some other chronic skin condition. I'm a skin cancer specialist, so many of my patients come to me because they are concerned about a spot on their body. Often, for a patient in his or her thirties or forties, this is their first dermatologic appointment ever. I ask them what brought them in, and they tell me that they noticed a brown spot that's getting bigger. Most of the time it turns out to be a seborrheic keratosis, or sun spot. But they did their due diligence and came in. I look them over, head to toe, and usually the news is good. Sometimes it's not so good, but in that case it is even better to get checked out so we can spot a problem before it becomes more dangerous.

Q: What is the first appointment like? What happens during a skin exam?

A: In the examining room, you will be asked to take all your clothes off and put on a gown that is open in the front. (There's no need to feel embarrassed; we doctors are used to doing this every day. But if you feel uncomfortable in any way, ask to have a nurse or doctor's assistant in the room during the exam. And if you feel nervous about baring it all, you may decline—although this defeats the purpose of a total body skin check.) You should take off your socks, your underwear, any hair bands, and your jewelry. Expect the dermatologist to look at your skin everywhere, starting at your head. I look through the scalp, behind and in the ears, on the face. I look under eyebrow hairs, on the eyelids, into the eyes and nose, and inside the mouth. I check the lymph nodes, scan the underarms, and look at the hands, between the fingers, on the nails. I go down the front of the body, including the groin area, down to the feet, in between the toes, to the nails and the soles of the feet. Then I take a look at the back side of the body. I lightly touch the skin the entire time I'm doing a skin check, feeling for little bumps or lumps along the way. Some doctors may have a patient lie down during the examination, but more often you will be standing up. The doctor may use a special magnifying glass or a Wood's lamp (or black light) to better observe a certain area or spot. Some dermatologists are faster and some are slower with their skin checks, but what is important is the thoroughness of the exam.

When I mention that dermatologists see lots of naked skin on a daily basis, I'm not exaggerating. We see brown spots, red marks, abnormal lesions, and sun spots hundreds of times a week. We are trained to detect a suspicious lesion, and at some point, we have a sixth sense of what's bad and what's normal. The problem is that a lot of skin cancers mimic benign-looking things such as freckles, scars, or skin tags. That puts some of the responsibility on you to look at your own skin from head to toe and be aware of any changes. Ask your doctor to show you how to do a skin self-exam.

Q: How can I do a skin check at home, and how often do I need to do it?

A: We should all give our skin a once-over every month. (I recommend doing your self-check on the day of your birthday. It's an easy way to remember.) Most of us don't do it at all. The truth is, I'm also guilty of forgetting or not bothering. But if you catch something early, it can save your life. You don't really have to know exactly what you're looking for. Just know your own skin. If something has changed, the computer system in your mind is going to notice. That's all you need to tell your doctor, and that's enough. It is incredibly helpful just to bring our attention to it.

The best time to do a skin self-exam is when you get out of the shower, as you're drying yourself off in the bathroom. There's usually a mirror in there, and you'll have some privacy and probably three minutes to spare. Examine your body front and back in the mirror, then look at the right and left sides with your arms raised. Look at your arms, inside your arms and your hands. Inspect your legs, front, and back, your feet, between the toes, and on the soles. If you have a hand mirror, try to check inside your ears, look behind your ears, on your back, on your scalp. Comb through your hair and use a hair dryer to blow it to the sides and inspect your scalp in as many areas as possible.

Enlist help too. If possible, ask your partner to check hard-to-see places such as your back. But do it together while you look in the mirror, so you can see too. (You can check his or her skin out too, while you're at it.) When you get your hair done, ask your hairstylist if he or she sees any spots on your scalp. Your dentist should do a skin cancer check inside your mouth as part of your regular checkup. Your eye doctor should check for skin cancer, and your gynecologist should too. Ask them.

Q: What happens if the doctor spots something suspicious? Does the patient get a biopsy that day?

A: If you need a biopsy, I like to take care of it immediately and get it over with that day, depending on how involved it might be. There are different methods used to obtain a sample for a pathologist, and some are less invasive than others. No matter which manner of biopsy your dermatologist chooses, it should take no longer than a few minutes. You get the results of a biopsy within a week by phone. (I will go into greater detail about biopsies in the next chapter on skin cancer.)

DID YOU CHECK...?

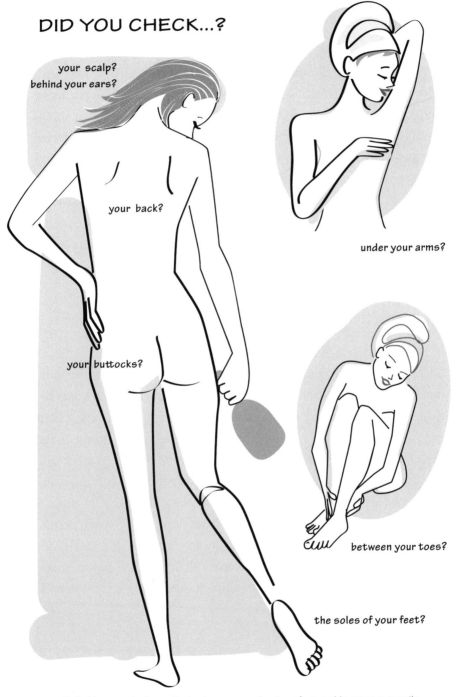

your scalp?
behind your ears?

your back?

your buttocks?

under your arms?

between your toes?

the soles of your feet?

Self skin examination—look at every centimeter of your skin once a month.
Have a partner look at your skin too.

Q: What personal or medical information should I be prepared to give my dermatologist?

A: You will have to fill out a medical intake form upon your first visit. A lot of the usual patient history questions will be asked on the form: Do you have any allergies? Do you have a family history of skin cancer? Have you ever had skin cancer before? Be sure to fill out these forms completely and accurately, because doctors read them carefully and they are very important. But dermatology is such a visual field that we don't always need to know an extensive personal history because we can look at the skin and recognize patterns. You may be asked specific questions, such as: How long have you had this spot? Has it changed? What treatments have you had?

Q: What other advice do you have for first-time patients?

A: During an average appointment, a doctor has approximately ten to fifteen minutes to spend with a patient. Studies have shown that doctors who accept medical insurance have only seven minutes per patient. You want to make the most of your time, but don't expect your dermatologist to be able to cover more than three issues on the initial visit. First and foremost, at that first appointment, I want to make sure you don't have skin cancer. If a patient overwhelms me with too many issues and questions all at the same time, I'm more likely to make a mistake in interpreting information. Please don't expect your dermatologist to be able to answer all your questions about skin care products, cosmetic treatments, and skin cancer all in the same appointment. You may need more than one appointment. Plus, that's what this book is for!

>>> **A REAL PATIENT STORY:**
Mixing Cosmetic with Medical Procedures

This account doesn't concern one particular patient. Instead, it illustrates a phenomenon that happens frequently with *many* of my patients. They ask me for Botox injections right after they've had a biopsy or while they are in skin cancer surgery. This happens about five times a week. And I can't say I blame them. (Being a multitasker myself, I'd probably do the same thing.) People would much rather be in my office for a voluntary cosmetic procedure than scary medical issues, and they consider their request to be an efficient use of time. There they are, already having something traumatic done, so why not shoot another needle or two into the skin at the same time? I tell patients that as a dermatologist my job is medical first. During surgery, whether it is a simple biopsy or a cancer excision, I want to concentrate clearly on the problem at hand. It's better to make an appointment for a cosmetic consultation later, so I can give the surgery issues my full attention. It's important that your dermatologist not be sidetracked, whether doing a biopsy or surgery, administering cosmetic filler, or performing an exam.

A patient interrupting a skin exam by asking too many cosmetic questions is also a common occurrence. Before I begin, I give patients an opportunity to tell me about any areas they are concerned about and to show me those spots. As I begin the exam, I have a clean map of the body in my mind; every centimeter of the skin is part of that map. As I perform the examination, I'm drawing on that map in my mind—there's a red spot on the left parietal scalp, a brown spot on the right bottom earlobe. I'm holding all that information in my memory until I can fill out the data on paper that I was visually taking in. (Sometimes there is an assistant in the room who writes down my oral notes, but often doctors don't have a "scribe" in the room.) In a single moment I may have seen a dysplastic nevus (an irregular brown spot) that looks worrisome. I'm focusing on how serious I think the spot is and what method of biopsy I should choose. If at that moment the patient is asking me questions about Botox or laser hair removal or which sunscreen I recommend, I am likely to make an error. It's better to let your doctor finish the assessment and explain it to you before asking cosmetic questions, even if you have to make a separate consultation appointment. It's tough to shift gears, and I find that I'm a much better doctor if I separate the two.

7

Skin Cancer

My Skin Cancer

My nicknames at Vassar College were "Nature Girl" and "Ivory Girl." The latter might have had something to do with the color of my complexion: ivory pale, a classic Fitzpatrick Type 1. I was the all-American girl—fresh-faced, freckled, and fair-skinned. Growing up in Happy Valley, Pennsylvania, I was an admitted tomboy—a swimmer, a cyclist, an outdoor athlete. And remember I led those canoeing trips in the Canadian wilderness for a couple of years. I was always outside in the sun and certainly didn't slather on sunscreen as I do now.

I was thirty-seven years old and five months pregnant with my second child when I was diagnosed with skin cancer. It was May 2006. I had pregnancy acne and noticed a little pink pimple—a smooth, pearly pink bump—on the right side of my nose. It wouldn't go away and never came to a head, and after a week or two, I had a feeling it wasn't normal. I showed it to my friend Dr. Leonard Bernstein, who had been one of my mentors at Cornell during my residency, and asked him to do a biopsy. Ironically, a few days later I had just finished filming a television interview about skin cancer awareness when Leon called. "El, you've got a skin cancer." Leon is the kind of guy who plays practical jokes all the time, so I was laughing at first. Then he said, "No, Ellen, really, it's basal cell carcinoma. You've got basal cell carcinoma, El." I remember being stunned. Everything stopped. Time stopped, sound stopped, and I thought, "Oh my God, I have skin cancer." It was an existential moment, within a nanosecond, life started again and my next thought was "Okay, I'll take care of it." I coped. As a skin cancer surgeon, I knew exactly what had to be done, so I set it up immediately.

Within forty-eight hours of the diagnosis I definitely had my first midlife crisis. I knew that the cancer I had was curable, but it was the first chink in my armor. It showed me that my physical body could break down. It's scary, because suddenly you know you don't have control over every cell in your body. If this is happening on my skin, what else is happening on the inside? I always trusted that my body was healthy and in balance, and now I suddenly understood that I was vulnerable. I also knew that once a person gets one skin cancer, he or she is at much higher risk (twenty-five times higher) of making others, including melanoma. (Arizona Senator John McCain, for example had both basal cell *and* squamous cell cancers after the surgical removal of malignant melanomas. The fair-skinned senator has had an unfortunate and extensive history of sun damage, including five years being held captive outdoors as a POW during the Vietnam War.)

I had Mohs micrographic surgery two days after my diagnosis. (Again, ironically, I specialize in this surgery.) Mohs is a minimally invasive surgery done for nonmelanoma skin cancers such as basal cell carcinoma (BCC) and squamous cell carcinoma (SCC). The procedure is done in stages and involves removing the cancerous lesion, checking the tissue under a microscope to see if all the margins are clean of cancer, and, if necessary, excising more of the abnormal tissue and checking again until the section is free of cancer. The surgery is done in one day, and the patient waits one to two hours in between the stages while the doctor processes the pathology. Because of its supreme accuracy Mohs surgery has a 99.9 percent cure rate, and since it spares more healthy tissue, it leaves a much smaller scar than regular surgery. (I will discuss Mohs surgery in more depth later in this chapter.)

My surgery took two stages, since in the first stage the pathology showed that there was still cancer in the margin (the border between healthy and abnormal tissue). That was another shocker. It was a surreal experience—as I imagine it is for most of my patients with skin cancer. To make matters even more surreal, I looked at my own skin cancer tissue under the microscope. It took about six months for my nose to heal, but I could be sure that I was free of BCC in that area. Basal cell carcinoma usually stays within the top couple layers of the skin and doesn't spread to other areas unless it has been there for a long time. When my doctor checked the margins, he also gauged the depth of the lesion. This type of cancer (like squamous cell carcinoma) tends to grow contiguously, meaning it grows as one big lesion, like a tree with roots. There are no disconnected spots scattered around like shrapnel that can get into the bloodstream and cause the cancer to spread unless it's very advanced.

Two years later, I'm healthy and fine (with a happy, beautiful baby girl, I might add). Last year I found a little brown dot on my knee, and when it turned darker the same red alert went off in my mind. I had it surgically excised and biopsied, and it turned out to be a premelanoma. Do I need to tell you again how important it is to do self–skin checks? I can say from personal experience that being aware of changes on your skin (and not ignoring them) can save your life.

When I walk into the examination room to consult with a patient who is about to have a biopsy or has a skin cancer that needs to be removed, I know how scared he or she is. (I was terrified myself.) Patients don't know what's going to happen; they think they're going to be deformed by the surgery. So I walk in and immediately tell them that I had skin cancer too and show them exactly where mine was taken off. I can feel the relief in their sigh. Then I begin to explain to them how we're going to tackle their particular skin cancer.

Skin cancer is by far the most prevalent cancer in the United States, with more than one million new cases diagnosed this year, and that number is rising by almost 5 percent annually. That accounts for half of all new cancer cases each year. Current estimates are that one in five Americans will develop skin cancer in their lifetime. Melanoma is the deadliest form, accounting for more than 75 percent of skin cancer deaths. The single biggest risk factor for most skin cancers is sun exposure, which causes 90 percent of them. The fact that these skin cancer numbers are rising means that something is obviously wrong. We're not getting the message somehow—about wearing sunscreen, about getting skin exams, about protecting ourselves from a cancer that is one of the most preventable. Skin cancers that are caught early are 98 to 100 percent curable, yet most adults have never been checked for skin cancer by a dermatologist. In a 2004 survey of 190 college students, less than 6 percent had ever checked their entire body for skin cancer. The National Cancer Institute reports that only 56 percent of adults say they protect themselves from the sun. That is as shocking a fact as the five that follow.

Five Shocking Facts About Skin Cancer

1. Melanoma is the most common cancer in young adults.

Melanoma is the most common form of cancer in people aged 25 to 29 and second (to Hodgkin's lymphoma) in adolescents and young adults ages 15 to 29.[1] A new study, published in the *Journal of Investigative Dermatology*, reports that melanoma rates in young women age 15 to 39 have soared 50 percent since 1980. In women 30 to 34 years old, breast cancer is most common, followed closely by melanoma. Why are younger people at higher risk? It's believed that the parallel rise in the use of tanning salons and sunbathing by teens is to blame. Many studies show that even though they are educated about the dangers of sun exposure and there are better sunscreens on the market, most teenagers and twenty-somethings either are numb to the message or believe they won't be the one in five who gets skin cancer.

I met a beautiful young woman with a golden tan who told me she goes to a tanning bed every week. I couldn't resist warning her about the danger she was in. Her reaction was far from shock or surprise. She guiltily gave me a laundry list of tanning justifications: "I only tan once a week. It's the only bad thing I do. I'm only in there for eight minutes. It doesn't give you a burn, just a tan." She told me that she wears sunblock dutifully and does regular self–skin checks. "I'm very careful about my skin," she added without an ounce of irony. "Besides, tanning makes me feel and look better, it's pretty. I'm still young, I'm only twenty two." This is an intelligent girl, but she has no intention of stopping her weekly tanning habit. Her contradictory actions and explanations are confounding, but she's obviously not alone. According to tanning industry estimates, approximately 28 million Americans are using some form of indoor tanning annually, and this could have an influence on those rising numbers. Even occasional use of tanning beds triples the chances of developing melanoma. The incidence of sunburns in teens and people in their twenties is higher than ever. In a nationwide survey done by the American Academy of Dermatology in 2005, almost 80 percent of teens said they knew tanning was dangerous and could increase their risk of skin cancer. Sixty-six percent believed that people look better and healthier with a tan, and 60 percent admitted that they had gotten sunburned that summer. Perhaps they feel invincible, as we all did in our teens and twenties. Nevertheless, this denial is clearly a very dangerous trend.

2. Not all skin cancers are sun-related, and some don't happen on the skin.

It's a fact that sun exposure is the primary cause of most skin cancers, providing the one-two punch of creating DNA mutations and suppressing the immune system. But other factors play a role too. Genetics contributes to the development of melanoma, even though approximately 65 percent of melanomas are attributed to UV radiation. Because sun exposure triggers immunosuppression over the entire body, it can create skin cancers anywhere—not just in local areas that receive direct sun. Many can begin where the sun doesn't shine like the mouth. Oral cancer starts on the wet mucosal areas, such as the palate, where there's no stratum corneum. It can look like a white or a red patch or a brown spot. (Your dentist probably checks for skin cancer during a regular exam, but be sure to ask.) Squamous cell carcinoma is the most common skin cancer in the mouth, and the chronic burns and carcinogens from cigarette smoking put smokers at higher risk (although 25 percent of oral cancers occur in nonsmokers). SCC can also occur in the nasal passages and in the genital area.

Skin cancers of the eye usually do stem from sun exposure. (Ultraviolet light actually penetrates through the full thickness of the lid, so it can generate cancer on the underneath part near the eyeball.) Any malignancy around the eye can invade along your eyeball if it spreads. Uveal melanoma, in the iris, is actually the number one source of metastatic melanoma from an unknown primary source. If someone has melanoma that has spread to the lungs and other organs and we can't find the source on the skin, it usually started in the eye. Melanoma starts in the uvea, where melanocytes generate your eye color. The incidence of uveal melanoma, just like that of other cancers, is highest among people with light skin and light eyes. It is a terrific reason to wear broad-spectrum UV-protective sunglasses.

Suffice it to say that skin cancers can show up in surprising, hidden places: on the soles of the feet, on the palms of the hands, under the nails, on the scalp, inside the ears, in the genital area, in the mouth, in the belly button and in the eye. Being vigilantly alert to any changes *anywhere* on your skin is vital.

3. *Having dark skin does not shield you from skin cancer.*

Darker skin types are definitely more protected against sun-induced skin cancer because of the production of melanin, but they are not immune. I have one patient, a woman with dark Type 5 skin, who's had multiple basal cell carcinomas on her face. I just operated on another woman, also a Type 5, who has melanoma on her breast and a fourteen-year-old girl with Type 5 skin and a melanoma on her arm. Perhaps it's genetics or simply bad luck that made these people vulnerable. (Admittedly, the first two women were major sun worshipers, so whether the sun crippled their immune systems from fighting off the cancer is another argument.) Acral lentiginous melanoma (ALM), which is often found on the hands and feet, accounts for 5 percent of diagnosed melanoma cases in the United States. It is the most common form of melanoma in Asians, African Americans, and dark-skinned populations. ALM is one of those hidden cancers—besides the palms and soles, it can lurk in overlooked spots like the mucous membranes of the nose or mouth, in the genital area and under toe and fingernails. Many people with dark skin who get skin cancers are diagnosed at a later stage, when the disease is more aggressive and potentially deadly. Although fewer African Americans develop skin cancer, a larger number of them die of the disease because it's not detected in time. In 1981, the reggae legend Bob Marley died of acral lentiginous melanoma that started underneath his right big toenail. Tragically, he mistook it for a soccer injury and ignored it until it spread to his lungs and brain. He was only thirty-six years old.

4. *There are more than one hundred different kinds of skin cancer.*

There are as many different kinds of cancer as there are types of cells in the skin. The mind reels with the frightening (although much more uncommon) possibilities. Most skin cancers are linked to sun exposure and immunosuppression. Merkel cell carcinoma, for example, is a rare but aggressive skin cancer that starts in the neuroendocrine cells called Merkel cells. These cells work with the nervous system and make the skin sensitive to the touch. There are approximately 1,200 new cases of Merkel cell carcinoma diagnosed in the United States every year, compared with almost 60,000 new cases of melanoma and over one million cases of nonmelanoma skin cancers. I see about one or two cases a year. Angiosarcoma is another cancer, which begins in the lining of the blood vessels. It can arise anywhere but often originates in the dermis of the skin. Cancers can develop in the fat cells of the skin and one, dermatofibrosarcoma protuberans or DFSP, in the fibroblast cells that make collagen. DFSP is an aggressive cancer that can track the whole dermal level of the skin and spread quickly. I see this about ten times a year, and its appearance on the skin mimics a scar—a little, hard, tan bump (similar to the nick you get from shaving). If something like this grows, changes, or just does not go away, please have it looked at by a doctor. Too often, when symptoms of these cancers appear on the skin, it's already advanced. Indeed, a cancer that begins somewhere inside the body can migrate to the skin. Usually metastasis on the skin is nodular—something you can feel as well as see, like a little line of marbles under the surface.

5. Children can get melanoma too.

Melanoma can—and does—occur in every age group. It is uncommon, but children do get skin cancer. Unfortunately, warning signs are missed because most people think that it's not possible for children to develop the disease. Pediatric melanoma is rare (making up only 2 percent of all melanomas). It affects only seven in 1 million children and adolescents, according to 2002 statistics from the National Cancer Institute. But that number has increased steadily since 1982, when the number was three per million children. Proper diagnosis is frequently overlooked because children often have a few little brown or reddish brown spots, called Spitz nevi. They look completely normal and are usually benign moles or birthmarks, but sometimes they can become early melanomas. Although there is little research currently available, it is believed that genetic predisposition can be a strong factor in these cases. The way a person's DNA deck of cards is shuffled can make him or her much more prone to melanoma mutations and tumor genesis due to sun exposure. In many cases of pediatric melanoma, the patients did not have traditional high-risk factors (fair skin and light eyes or a family history of the disease). One thing is sure: they all had moles that changed or appeared atypical. This is something a parent should watch for and an important reason to see a dermatologist for an annual checkup—even as a child.

>>> **A REAL PATIENT STORY:**
Skin Cancers Masquerade as Other Things

A simple cosmetic procedure has frequently led me to detect something serious. Recently a good friend of mine came in for a laser treatment to get rid of some sun damage and brown spots. As I was inspecting the areas to laser, I noticed something suspicious on her neck—a white-pink, flat spot that appeared to be a scar. She said it had been there for years, but I asked if I could take a biopsy. My philosophy as a doctor is always to put medicine first, so I biopsied that area, then laser-treated the other spots she had originally come in for. That spot turned out to be basal cell carcinoma. I just performed Mohs surgery, and she's going to be absolutely fine.

About once every other week, a patient comes in for cosmetic laser treatment to get rid of a few brown spots and one of them triggers my sixth sense. It's usually a light tan, flat freckle that may be slightly darker or larger than the others or a little bit scaly. I always ask to biopsy something like this *before* I do any kind of cosmetic procedure. Patients have different reactions. Most are very agreeable and have a biopsy. One man came in to laser off a brown sun-damaged area on his chest and I biopsied one atypical brown spot. It was diagnosed as a severely dysplastic nevus (which is premelanoma), and he dodged a big bullet. Another woman saw me for laser treatment, and I was concerned about one particularly large brown mark on her cheek. When I suggested a biopsy, she got very angry and told me that other doctors had seen it and she'd had it for years. "Why would you need to do a biopsy? I just came in for laser treatment. Now I'm nervous." I assured her that I just wanted to make sure that it wasn't something serious before I did an elective cosmetic procedure. Hers was benign, and I could safely do laser on the lesion in good conscience. "Better safe than sorry" is always the best dermatologic motto in my practice.

On the other hand, I've examined patients with something I thought was benign—a fleshy growth or a small scaly patch—and I've taken it off. Whenever I remove any tissue from the skin, I always send it out for pathology. (Most doctors do this; insurance should cover the pathology, and patients should insist on it.) One time, tissue that I believed was benign came back as basal cell carcinoma. I was completely wrong. A colleague of mine removed some skin tags from a patient, sent them for pathology as routine procedure, and it was melanoma. We are trained skin cancer specialists, and these things can deceive even us. This is why your personal sixth sense about changes in your own skin is so very important.

How Skin Cancer Begins

Cancer is a case of normal cells going bad and then growing at an alarming rate. This population of abnormal cells becomes more and more massive until they take over resources of blood supply and nutrients. It's an unchecked revolution in your body. "Oncogenesis" is the medical name for this process of transformation that occurs when healthy cells become malignant. In skin cancer it begins with UV radiation causing DNA damage, which in turn causes all kinds of genes to be triggered. For example, there is a specific gene (the P53 tumor suppressor gene) whose job is to regulate the cell growth cycle and to stop tumors. This gene is like an intelligence spy in the field. When it spots something wrong, P53 calls on other genes to create a cell-cycle blockade to stop the growth of the cell so the DNA can be repaired. If a cell has been damaged beyond repair, P53 can induce apoptosis, or programmed cell death. The damaged cell basically commits suicide, shutting down forever. ("Apoptosis" comes from a Greek word meaning "leaves falling off trees," and the same thing happens here, genetically.) This prevents the retention of mutations. If a cell can't stop to fix its DNA damage, that cell will make a new population of mutated cells, and that is cancer. If the P53 gene, the guardian of the DNA program or genome, is traumatized by sun damage, a mutant population of cells can proliferate. Skin cancers usually occur after years of cumulative sun damage has inactivated P53 tumor suppressor genes, disarmed the immune system, and generated mutant populations of cells that now can grow out of control.

Are You at High Risk?

If you have fair skin (Fitzpatrick Types 1, 2, or 3) with light hair and light eyes, you are at high risk. If you have a family history of skin cancer or have had a skin cancer (or any other cancer) in the past, you are at high risk. If you have more than fifty moles on your body, you are at high risk. If you are a smoker or frequent tanning beds, your chances of getting skin cancer are greatly increased. If you spend a majority of your time outdoors or have had a lot of sun damage, you are at very high risk, and if you don't use sunscreen regularly, you've put yourself in double jeopardy. The problem with talking about increased risk is that the people who aren't tagged as high risk think they are safe and don't protect themselves or get skin checks. Anyone with skin is in danger of developing skin cancer. That's why we *all* need to be on our guard with sunscreen and skin checks.

Detecting Skin Cancer

I cannot stress strongly enough the importance of early detection. Skin cancer has a high cure rate if it's caught early and treated correctly. Squamous cell carcinoma and basal cell carcinoma have a five-year cure rate of 97 to 99 percent. This means that the recurrence rate after five years is extremely low. So there is no reason to panic if you have a small skin cancer that is diagnosed early. Because they stay localized in one area, it can take years for these kinds of cancers to spread. But if a lesion is not removed or treated, it is going to grow and it will spread. I have seen ten cases of metastatic basal cell carcinoma in my relatively young career. It is rare but extremely devastating, and it can be lethal. I've seen approximately one hundred cases of metastatic squamous cell carcinoma. If melanoma is caught early, it is 100 percent curable. If the tumor is slightly invasive but still contained to the top levels of the skin, there's a 95 percent five-year cure rate. Catching melanoma at an early stage is more common than ever before, thanks to improved awareness about sun damage and skin cancer. The public is more educated and much more aware of warning signs on their skin.

In patients who are high risk of melanoma or if a patient points out an irregular dark spot or lesion (an atypical nevus, or mole), I use my trained clinical eye and the assistance of technology to take a closer look and better distinguish between a benign or dysplastic (malignant) nevus. These diagnostic tools are used to photograph and get a microscopic look at a pigmented area of skin that could turn out to be malanoma. They also help doctors gauge how large a lesion is and how deep it might be in the skin.

Wood's Lamp

A Wood's lamp is a handheld ultraviolet "black" light that enhances the appearance of pigmented lesions. It helps reveal melanomas at an early stage. This is the same kind of light used in spas (the one that makes your face appear to be a map of sun damage). To my naked eye, a lesion on someone's face might seem to be only the size of a dime, but when I hold a Wood's lamp to it I can see that it has spread all over the cheek—well beyond what I thought were the original margins. The limitation of the Wood's lamp is that it cannot evaluate depth of pigment, which determines how advanced a melanoma has become. (Most melanomas grow radially first, like an oil slick, and then begin to go down deeper into the skin.)

Dermoscopy

A dermatoscope is a handheld device that uses polarized light to magnify an area ten times. The features of a brown spot become more prominent and the pattern of pigment can be seen clearly (lesions may look gray, blue, red, or black under the dermatoscope). Most important, dermoscopy helps evaluate the depth of pigment. Most lesions that might be (or become) melanomas are almost always surgically removed for biopsy. But this strategy can prove problematic if there are multiple atypical lesions. The decision to biopsy all of them to see if they are indeed malignant could be disfiguring. At the same time, a doctor doesn't want to overlook something that could turn out to be malignant. Dermatologists have struggled with this dilemma for many years, and new technologies such as dermoscopy allow us to better evaluate a lesion while it's still in the body. Sometimes a lesion may appear atypical at first; then dermoscopy reveals it to be a simple angioma, a benign growth made up of blood vessels. This can prevent doing a biopsy. In other situations dermoscopy can give a doctor more confidence that a biopsy is absolutely necessary.

Mole Mapping

This digital imaging system uses a dermatoscope with the capability of taking magnified photographs of a lesion. I can then download the images to a computer program that evaluates its features and grades them. Mole mapping photographically documents quadrants of the body and allows me to monitor lesions, using the digital imaging to compare and identify changes in the skin. A patient is photographed one initial time; then I refer back to the photos when I examine him or her in the future, literally comparing what I see on the skin to what I see in the image. If I notice a new mole that does not exist in the photo album or any mole that's changed or appears unusual, I use a dermatoscope to take a detailed look or attach a camera to the instrument and take a magnified picture.

Most existing moles don't transform into melanoma. Usually it's new moles that you need to worry about. One study found that less than 5 percent of existing nevi become malignant, and of that minority of moles, the modifications were so subtle that most patients never detected them.[2] This certainly underscores the value of regular dermatologic checkups with digital dermoscopy for high-risk patients. In general, if a mole or spot hasn't changed in three months, 99 percent of the time it's not malignant. This is a good guideline but not complete security. I've been witness to that 1 percent malignancy too. To be safe, close monitoring and regular dermoscopy are a good line of defense.

New high-tech instruments are further advancing the state of melanoma surveillance. Confocal microscopy is a newly developed technique that allows us to visualize skin in microscopic detail and depth and high resolution. Another new digital photography system called MelaFind provides higher resolution and may turn out to be a superior magnifier to other digital dermoscopy devices. And three-dimensional imaging, which could help make diagnoses even more accurate, is under development. As amazing and state of the art as this technology is, it only aids a doctor's good judgment and sixth sense. It's the combination of medical know-how—the art of medicine, if you will—and these extraordinary tools that provide the key to a swift and accurate diagnosis.

If a doctor finds something suspicious, the next step is usually a biopsy—removal of part, or sometimes all, of the atypical tissue to be examined under a microscope. Biopsy is a scary word, but the procedure isn't too painful; it takes only a few minutes and doesn't leave a big scar. The patient is given a shot of lidocaine, a local anesthetic, to numb the area first, and then one of the following forms of biopsy is done, depending on the type of cancer we suspect it might be and the amount of skin we need to take. It takes approximately one week to get the results of a biopsy, and they are typically given over the phone.

Biopsy Methods

SHAVE

This is a minimally invasive biopsy. We use a flexible surgical blade to do a very superficial, paper-thin section of the lesion. (For lack of a better image, this is a bit like a cheese slicer that cuts a perfect, sheer circle of Parmesan.) This slice of tissue provides the pathologist a bigger sample to read. Sometimes I elect to do a "deep shave" biopsy on an area I suspect to be melanoma, scooping out a deeper sample of tissue to examine.

CURETTE

This method employs a tool with a small open circle on one end that is sharp on one side. One limitation is that curetting might provide a smaller specimen. Sometimes the pathologist can't get a sufficient view of the smaller sample of skin.

PUNCH

This technique uses a device that has a circular open tip with a sharp edge (it looks similar to a ballpoint pen). The doctor presses the punch into the skin and swivels it from side to side, removing a small but deep cylindrical core of tissue (rather than just the top part of skin). So there is a layer-cake specimen with the epidermis on top, the dermis in the middle, and fat underneath that. Because this enables the pathologist to read the depth of a lesion, a punch biopsy is done on a pigmented lesion that's suspected to be melanoma (where depth is the most important characteristic). Punch biopsies are limited to an area of skin that's only six to eight millimeters in diameter; for a larger lesion I would probably opt for an excision.

EXCISION

The entire tumor, including the borders of healthy tissue that surround it, is surgically removed. Although this is obviously the most invasive biopsy procedure, it is the best way to test for melanoma and excise the abnormal area at the same time. It is usually outpatient surgery done with a local anesthetic. The excision plus the stitches afterward take about thirty minutes, although a larger lesion obviously takes longer.

>>> skin lie: Biopsies can spread cancer.

>>> skin truth: A lot of people believe the myth that if you biopsy an area, you can disrupt the tumor and allow mutations to spread. This is untrue. But the entire premise of my field, Mohs micrographic surgery, is based on the misconception that it's dangerous to excise cancers. In 1936, Dr. Frederick E. Mohs created the innovative surgery as a response to this fear. With this technique, the surgeon has microscopic control as he or she removes abnormal tissue. When the tumor is removed, the surgeon processes the pathology, checks the margins right away, and, if need be, goes back and removes any malignant tissue that's left. (In standard surgery, the doctor must take wider margins, removing as much potentially dangerous tissue as possible just to be on the safe side, since the margins can't be checked with a microscope during the process.) When Mohs was originally done, the process utilized zinc chloride as a safe fixative that could be applied directly to the tissue that was being excised. It was painful, but this made the tissue solid, so it could be removed without the fear of causing single cells to spread. (It also

provided the added benefit of being easier to process for pathology.) Modern Mohs surgery is performed without fixative applied directly to the patient, but it still makes it possible to process and examine the tissue immediately.

Mohs surgery (originally conceived of as the answer to the fear of biopsies) is considered the gold standard of first-line treatment for basal cell and squamous cell carcinomas of the head, neck, hands, feet, and groin. These are considered to be areas where skin-saving, minimalist surgery is more crucial.

The Three Main Types of Skin Cancer

There are more than one hundred different types of skin cancer, but three—basal cell carcinoma, squamous cell carcinoma, and melanoma—are the most common. This is how they are detected and treated.

Basal Cell Carcinoma (BCC)

This is the most common form of skin cancer, accounting for about 90 percent of skin cancers diagnosed each year, and it has the lowest risk of metastasis. Although it is slow to spread, it certainly may do so, and needs to be treated immediately. Because the tumor grows contiguously, once it is excised, the recurrence risk is very low. BCC is 95 to 100 percent curable when caught early. By the way, there's been a sharp rise in both basal cell and squamous cell carcinomas in women under the age of forty (like me). These numbers have increased fourfold in the last thirty years, according to the Skin Cancer Foundation.

RED FLAGS FOR BCC

The classic basal cell carcinoma resembles the one I had: a pearly pink bump, like a pimple that doesn't go away. It's slightly elevated and smooth. But sometimes BCC can show up as a smooth, flat white-pink scar (these are more aggressive) or a brown patch that resembles a freckle. BCC can be a dry, crusty spot, or it can be ulcerated and tend to bleed. Most are located on the face and neck—sun-exposed areas.

FIRST-LINE TREATMENT FOR BCC

Excision is the most effective way to treat almost all skin cancers. For basal cell and squamous cell carcinomas, Mohs micrographic surgery is the gold standard because of its accuracy and because it spares tissue and leaves much less scarring—especially important if the lesion is on the face or neck. (Any doctor can call himself or herself a Mohs specialist, but that is not always the case. It's important to make sure that the dermatologist doing the procedure is actually a fellowship-trained Mohs surgeon. It's wise to double-check on the official Mohs surgery Web site: www.mohscollege.org.)

Another option, surgically, is curettage—electrodessication of the area—which is basically scraping and burning the lesion off the skin. This is probably the most common procedure used to treat BCC and SCC that is not on the face or neck. First the area is numbed with lidocaine; then the doctor uses a curette to scrape off the skin deeply in the area of the lesion. The area is then burned with an electrical pen. This scraping and burning is repeated three times. The limitation of electrodessication and curettage is this: the doctor has no idea if he or she actually got all of the cancer, and now the patient will have a scar there that may mask any malignancy underneath it. Consequently, the chance of recurrence with this method is up to 50 percent (while Mohs has a 1 percent risk of relapse). In my opinion, Mohs surgery is always the best choice aesthetically and for accuracy, but it is very expensive and sometimes insurance companies won't cover it (unless the lesion is on the face, neck, hands and feet).

If I see a large area of sun damage that looks precancerous but is not necessarily skin cancer, I use adjuvant therapies such as chemotherapy creams or photodynamic therapy. I wouldn't use these therapies as a substitute for surgery on a cancerous lesion. Mohs surgery has a 99 percent cure rate for BCC and SCC, while adjuvant treatments provide anywhere from a 20 percent to an 80 percent cure rate. However, they are a great follow-up to surgery, and can prevent further skin cancers in the future.

COMBINATION AND ADJUVANT THERAPIES FOR BCC

Because basal cell carcinoma is so aggressive by the time it metastasizes, there are no good nonsurgical interventions. Radiation may be used for older patients who cannot tolerate surgery, and immunotherapy creams (see "Squamous Cell Carcinoma" below) may help treat thin BCC, although they are not as effective as excision.

RADIATION THERAPY

Radiation is an option for targeting areas that are difficult to treat with surgery and a common alternative for those who can't have surgery for some reason. Radiation energy damages and destroys genetic material in both normal and cancer cells, and while the normal cells recover the malignant cells die off. It usually requires twenty sessions, and the skin can become red, irritated, and even ulcerated from the treatments.

Squamous Cell Carcinoma (SCC)

This is the second most common skin cancer, and, like BCC, it is usually located on sun-exposed areas. It also tends to stay localized but may spread and its metastasis is much faster than that of basal cell carcinoma. Interestingly, men are twice as likely to develop squamous cell and basal cell carcinomas than women, according to the Skin Cancer Foundation.

RED FLAGS

Precancerous lesions for squamous cell carcinoma are called "actinic keratoses" (AKs). They look like a red or brown patch of sun damage. A suspicious area tends to be crusty and dry, and it may bleed. Though these lesions may not become cancerous, they have a good chance of being precursors of SCC. If treated early, however, AKs can be eliminated before becoming skin cancer. In my own scientific study, I found that it takes approximately two years for an actinic keratosis to progress to a squamous cell carcinoma.[3]

FIRST-LINE TREATMENT FOR SCC

As with all skin cancers, surgical excision is the best remedy for squamous cell carcinoma that has penetrated the basement membrane of the skin. As with BCC, Mohs surgery is the gold standard. Also as with BCC, an alternative for the removal of small, superficial lesions can be curettage and electrodessication (scraping and burning).

PREVENTATIVE AND ADJUVANT THERAPIES FOR SCC (AND FIRST-LINE TREATMENT FOR ACTINIC KERATOSES)

These treatments are used with surgery in patients at high risk for recurrence of SCC and instead of surgery for early, superficial (in situ) cancers (especially on large areas of sun-damaged skin). They are also used to treat actinic keratoses: dry, rough, scaly patches of skin that look like sun damage but can develop into squamous cell cancers. (Some studies have suggested that actinic keratoses can also give rise to basal cell carcinoma, but more research needs to be done. So far there are no known precancers for BCC.)

PHOTODYNAMIC THERAPY (PDT)

This treatment destroys skin cancer cells by using a powerful light source that activates a chemical solution on the skin. It's especially effective for treating a large area of sun damage with a field of early cancers that are clinically invisible. I use it on patients who've already had skin cancer and have a 50 percent chance of producing others.

First aminolevulinic acid (ALA) is applied to the skin. It is allowed to remain there for three hours, absorbing into highly metabolic cells (namely, cancer cells, which consume oxygen and nutrients faster than regular cells). Then the ALA solution is illuminated with an LED blue

light for about twenty minutes. The chemical reaction that occurs produces by-products called porphyrins that proceed to obliterate the
cancer cells. That phototoxic effect makes the skin red, swollen, and
irritated, then causes it to peel. Recovery from PDT takes about six to
ten days. Oddly enough, the worse the skin looks after treatment, the
better the results because local destruction of precancerous lesions
causes the irritation and trauma to the area. For patients who have had
skin cancer or a lot of sun damage and actinic keratoses, I recommend
getting PDT three times a year.

TOPICAL CHEMOTHERAPY

A prescription cream, 5-fluorouracil, destroys mutant cells and causes
an inflammatory reaction. It is applied to a precancerous area for approximately four to eight weeks Theoretically this is considered chemotherapy because it utilizes chemicals, but I think the term scares
people. (When I discuss treatment options with my patients, one out
of twenty immediately refuses to use these topical creams because they
are afraid of chemo-like side effects. The primary side effect of this
topical chemo is fatigue.) As with PDT, chemotherapy for SCC is approximately 85 percent effective. It is best for AKs but can be used for
thin, in situ SCC and BCC.

IMMUNOTHERAPY CREAM

A topical medicine called imiquimod is an immunomodulator. It is designed to both diagnose cancers and stimulate the body's immune
system to rev up an attack on malignant cells. This is a great option for
treating AKs, in situ SCC, or early-stage BCC or for someone who has
many early or precancerous lesions in one area. It could prevent a potentially disfiguring surgical procedure and can eradicate approximately 80 percent of precancers and early superficial skin cancers.

    Imiquimod is applied to an entire area of sun-damaged skin (the
forehead, for instance) for four to sixteen weeks. In that time, certain
spots may become red, indicating a cancerous lesion, since the redness

means that inflammatory cells are attacking in that particular place. Similar in theory to the immunotherapy used for melanoma, this treatment causes the body to recognize and mount an assault on mutant cells. Although they work in different ways, both of these topical therapies are used for the same end point: preventing precancers (or very superficial tumors on the surface of the skin) from becoming cancers or spreading. Unfortunately, the side effects of both medications can include itching, redness, blistering, flaking, and overall irritation.

PREVENTATIVE TREATMENT FOR ACTINIC KERATOSES ONLY

When I see a large area of actinic keratoses, I use a less invasive course of treatment on it. There are many effective therapeutic options, including topical immunotherapy, chemotherapy, and photodynamic therapy. A dermatologist will weigh the pros and cons with the patient. Some treatments (such as chemotherapy creams), can be done at home but will take weeks, and some are done in the office in one day but can require quite a bit of recovery time. Each method is a destructive modality and has its share of side effects, but all of them can prove effective at eliminating actinic keratoses and preventing them from turning into squamous cell cancer. There is no single perfect method, which is why my approach is combination therapy. Rather than one massive treatment, I use a little bit of everything and keep treating and monitoring the patient every three to six months until the lesions are all gone. If someone has one small lesion, I usually choose to excise it or use liquid nitrogen on the spot. But if there are many red, scaly areas (called a field effect), treating them is going to be a three-times-a-year cycle of therapies to get the damage to slowly go away.

CHEMICAL PEELS

Many precancers, such as actinic keratosis, are in the epidermis. Because they are on the surface of the skin, fairly invasive chemical peels such as a 30% trichloracetic acid (TCA) peel and also fractionated laser or CO_2 laser resurfacing of the skin can take them off. These methods literally burn off the damaged cells, along with the top surface of the skin. (Laser resurfacing is more expensive and not often used as a treatment for AKs.) Both treatments have been shown to decrease the incidence of squamous cell precancers. TCA is also melanotoxic, which means it decimates melanosomes (tiny balloons containing melanin), so it works well on pigment problems such as melasma. Frequently, I treat a section of sun-damaged actinic keratosis with a TCA peel spot treatment, rather than treating the entire face and neck. After a peel like this, the patient's skin becomes red and irritated, and after a day or two the damaged stratum corneum starts to peel off. Ironically, it looks and feels like a horrible sunburn.

CRYOSURGERY

This is a common treatment for actinic keratoses utilizing liquid nitrogen (the same chemical that makes dry ice) in a freezing cold spray. It works with the freeze-thaw cycle: the spray freezes the abnormal cells; then, as they thaw, the cells expand and explode. This can effectively spot treat small lesions. Cryotherapy is very painful and can leave white scars where the pigment has been blasted by liquid nitrogen. For this reason, I don't use it for removing precancers as much as I do a TCA peel spot treatment.

FOLLOW-UP TREATMENT FOR BCC AND SCC

For any skin cancer, the patient must see the dermatologist in three months for a skin exam. If you are clear of basal cell or squamous cell carcinoma in that time, the doctor will probably ask to see you again in six months. If at that time you are cancer-free, an annual exam will be fine. But all patients should be checking their own skin and protecting themselves by staying out of the sun and wearing sunscreen every day, since the chance of developing any kind of skin cancer again is higher for them. Topical tretinoin, or retinoic acid, has also been prescribed to help prevent the recurrence of nonmelanoma skin cancers.

Melanoma

Although it accounts for only 4 percent of skin cancer cases, melanoma is the deadliest form of the disease. According to the American Cancer Society, one American dies of melanoma every hour. In 2008, 8,420 deaths will be attributed to this cancer—5,400 men and 3,020 women. While there are genetic links to the disease, sun exposure remains the biggest factor we can control. Indeed, the Skin Cancer Foundation has found that women who rarely use sunscreens have twice the melanoma risk of women who always wear sunscreen.

RED FLAGS FOR MELANOMA

Dermatologists look at nevi, which are moles. There are benign melanocytic nevi or normal moles, and dysplastic nevi, which have abnormal growth patterns. Doctors grade the latter as either mildly, moderately, or severely dysplastic. It's difficult to tell which ones might go on to become malignant, but severely dysplastic nevi are regarded as precancerous melanoma and are always surgically removed. (Many people may have thirty or more dysplastic nevi, and we can't excise them all without disfiguration. These are cases where dermoscopy and close monitoring are invaluable.) Almost all of the time, melanoma appears as a pigmented lesion, but it can sometimes show up as a pink bump or a vertical brown streak on a fingernail or toenail. It may look like a scar, or it may be a sore that bleeds all the time. The symptoms are very sneaky. As a rule, these are the warning signs that we should be on guard for, the ABCs (plus the D and E) of melanoma:

	A = Asymmetry	Because melanoma has a radial growth phase first, spreading like an oil slick, early melanomas do not look perfectly round like normal moles; they are asymmetric.
	B = Borders	A melanoma has indistinct edges that are hazy and smudgy, as if the border has been erased.
	C = Color	Multiple colors (such as blue, gray, black, or red) can represent malignancy. Red pigment may be a sign of inflammation or of angiogenesis (the growth of blood vessels to feed a tumor). If one pigmented lesion stands out as much darker than the others, that's a suspicious characteristic. This is known as "the ugly duckling sign." Dark blue, black, or gray pigment can signify that the nevus is dense and growing deeper into the skin. A disappearance of color can also be a sign of regression—a characteristic of aggressive malignant lesions.
	D = Diameter	Larger than six millimeters (about the size of a pencil eraser) is considered large—and dangerous.
	E = Elevation or evolving	If something that was flat quickly becomes elevated (becoming a nodular bump), that is a sign of tumor growth. Be aware of any existing mole that changes in some way or begins to bleed. (Ulceration is a signal that the malignancy is aggressive.)

The ABCDE's of atypical moles and melanomas.

FIRST-LINE TREATMENT FOR MELANOMA

The first-line treatment (the best plan of attack) for most skin cancers, especially melanoma, is surgery. For melanoma I always excise, although sometimes surgeons can do only a partial excision if the tumor is too large or affects an essential body part such as the spine, heart, or brain. Surgery for melanoma is much more invasive and extensive than excision of other skin cancers because the cancer grows vertically— deep down into the skin. Melanoma is like mold inside your walls; it seeps down deeply and can destroy anything in its path. For this reason, surgeons sometimes have to go past the fat layer of skin to the muscle in order to take out a tumor. It's also necessary to take wide margins to make sure the cancer hasn't leeched into healthy tissue nearby. Usually surgery for melanoma is an outpatient procedure, unless the area of skin to be excised is very large.

When a surgeon excises melanoma that is deeper than one millimeter, he or she always discusses the option to check to see if the lymph nodes are involved by doing a sentinel lymph node biopsy. If melanoma is detected there, the doctor usually surgically removes the cancerous nodes, then may also irradiate the area or propose adjuvant therapy. (This is considered Stage III melanoma.) Cancers can spread in the tissue, through the bloodstream, or in the lymph nodes (which are part of the circulatory system). Lymph vessels are spider web–delicate and course throughout the body. They act as a super-highway for immune cells. The lymph nodes, located in various areas—such as the underarms, groin, elbow area, and lungs—are like rest stops. At the core of each node is the germinal center, where immune cells are made, become specialized, and are released into the body to provide disaster relief where it's needed. When cancer invades the lymph nodes, it can obviously spread even faster on this super-highway. At this advanced stage, even with successful treatment, there is a 30 to 50 percent chance the cancer will recur.

If melanoma is superficial (in situ), meaning it's still contained to the top layers of skin and has not begun to invade deeper, Ruby laser treatment has been used to basically burn it off the skin. But this is usually done only if the lesion is large. As a rule, no treatment for skin cancer is as effective as surgery, and that is the method I would choose in almost any case. Anything on your skin that is proven to be malignant should be surgically removed if possible.

Another scary and insidious aspect of the way melanoma spreads (which is different from that of other skin cancers) is "single-cell metastasis," in which a mutant cell can get into the circulation, lodge itself someplace else, and start building a population there. Some of the adjuvant (or additional secondary) treatments for melanoma address the possibility of these rogue cells hiding somewhere in the body.

ADJUVANT THERAPIES FOR MELANOMA

Additional treatment is begun following surgery for melanoma if a patient is at high risk for recurrence. In Stage II, involving a very deep lesion, the risk of recurrence is 60 percent after five years, and if the disease has progressed further, to Stage III, that risk spikes to 75 percent. A recurrence involves residual cancer left in the body from the original tumor. It can recur locally (adjacent to the original area) or distally, meaning it has metastasized through the bloodstream or the lymph nodes. A secondary melanoma is a separate malignancy that pops up somewhere else, unrelated to the original melanoma. The following are the standard (and one experimental) adjuvant therapies associated with melanoma. All incur negative side effects (like nausea or fatigue), and each has its pros and cons. A dermatologist and oncologist will discuss the options in detail with a patient before setting forth on one of these therapeutic roads.

IMMUNOTHERAPY

This is standard treatment for metastatic melanoma after surgery. It utilizes interferon, the FDA-approved drug shown to improve survival rates in patients with a high rate of relapse. Interferon alpha-2b, given by infusions, is toxic to melanoma cells and works by encouraging the body's own immune system to recognize cancers and then fight them off. Side effects are extreme fatigue and flu-like symptoms.

CHEMOTHERAPY

Anticancer drugs, which are either taken orally or injected into the bloodstream, work to kill cancer cells. Chemotherapy is nonspecific, in that it kills malignant cells but is toxic to healthy cells too. There are more sophisticated chemotherapies being discovered that might be able to target specific melanoma cells by either blowing them up or inducing apoptosis, programmed cell death. As of now, there is no great chemotherapy for melanoma.

RADIATION

High doses of radiation take aim at melanoma in a specific area to destroy cancer cells. They are frequently used after surgery to double-treat a section. This method is frequently used on lymph nodes if surgery is not possible. It can be employed in conjunction with chemotherapy or used as a palliative treatment for advanced melanoma to relieve symptoms.

EXPERIMENTAL VACCINES

Many melanoma patients enroll in clinical trials that involve vaccines, or "nonspecific immunostimulants." (I worked on researching melanoma vaccines at New York University in 1999 with Dr. Jean-Claude Bystryn.) A vaccine teaches the body how to recognize and then attack a malignancy. Experimental melanoma vaccines can target the single rogue mutant cells that hide and set up shop somewhere in the body. Every single cell has a particular fingerprint that identifies what type it is, and this fingerprint takes the form of proteins. These vaccines try to get the body to identify the proteins found on melanoma cells, and then they kill the mutant cells. (Like other vaccines, they do this by using dead melanoma cells injected into the body, which will hopefully stimulate the immune system to attack.) The medical ramifications of a successful melanoma vaccine would be galvanizing. So far, however, such vaccines have not been effective for many patients as a way to fight off a recurrence of melanoma. Also, it is a painstaking process since the patient must receive a series of many injections over a span of many years.

Offering extraordinary promise for the future is a groundbreaking personalized vaccine that clones a patient's own fighter T-cells and infuses five billion of them back into that person's body. Because these immune cells are compatible, they are already educated to detect and kill that particular patient's melanoma. A study published in June 2008 in *The New England Journal of Medicine* showed that a man with advanced metastatic melanoma who was treated with this personalized vaccine had been cancer-free for two years.[4] The great success of this patient is encouraging and thrilling, but the effectiveness of this treatment still needs to be proven with further tests and in a larger study.

FOLLOW-UP TREATMENT FOR MELANOMA

After the original surgical treatment, most patients will need to see their dermatologist for a skin check every three months for one year. If they graduate to a low-risk level, they can come in every six months after that. Adjuvant therapies are continued until the patient is cured.

Experimental Therapies and Breakthrough Discoveries for the Future

We know how to help prevent skin cancer (stay out of direct sun and wear sunscreen!), and we have mainstream therapies that help to fight and eradicate the disease (surgery, chemotherapy, radiation, cryotherapy). There are also many other treatment options (PDT, TCA peels, immunotherapy) to inhibit it from recurring. And in this exciting day and age, a lot of fascinating, groundbreaking new treatments and preventive discoveries are being studied and perfected every day. I discussed the still-experimental melanoma vaccines that are being worked on and clinical trials for these are ongoing. Scientists are also working on new immune system–boosting drugs that can strengthen the body's own attack on cancer cells.

We seem to learn every week about a new antioxidant or magic pill that may help avert skin cancer. Though many of these new, "miraculous" discoveries should be taken with a grain of salt, some are being proven effective. Studies are being done to establish whether long-term use of aspirin and anti-inflammatory drugs such as ibuprofen can somehow lower the risk of nonmelanoma skin cancer and precancerous lesions. So far the jury is still out, and research is continuing. Many scientific studies have shown that the polyphenol antioxidants in green tea can help induce apoptosis in damaged cells. They have also been studied for their ability to inhibit urokinase, a protein produced by cancer cells that helps them invade healthy cells and spread. Resveratrol, the antioxidant in red wine and grapes, is being studied for its power to prevent DNA damage from the sun. Researchers are also investigating the anti–skin cancer potential of pomegranate extract, which has higher antioxidant activity than green tea or red wine. Whether these antioxidants work better when consumed in the diet or applied topically to the skin is still up in the air too. As scientists pursue these promising, novel ways to protect us from sun damage, the best prevention by far is what we already know works: broad-spectrum sunscreen and avoidance of direct UV radiation.

Interesting research is being done on a chemical called cyclopamine, derived from the corn lily plant. It has been shown to shrink BCC tumors in mice and inhibit new tumors by 90 percent.[5] Experimental testing is still being done on the cancer-fighting properties of barnacle-like marine animals called "tunicates." There is a compound, dubbed "palmerolide A," in the tunicate's biochemistry that may inhibit melanoma. Lab tests are still in the preliminary stages. Dimericine, a new topical cream, is in clinical trials and not yet approved by the FDA. It contains enzymes that help repair DNA damage. This could be effective as a treatment for actinic keratoses or to reduce non-melanoma skin cancers.

As exciting as all these experimental findings are, hope must be tempered with caution. There's no new wonder drug for skin cancer yet, and the gold standard treatment is still surgery.

More Information about Skin Cancer

I realize that this chapter provides just an overview of a very complex and serious subject. If you or someone you love is diagnosed with skin cancer, I recommend learning as much as you can and speaking honestly and openly with your dermatologist and oncologist. The following Web sites can prove a terrific starting point for research on various types of skin cancer and for learning more about how to prevent or treat the disease. They are an invaluable resource for those who want to find out about the latest research and experimental treatments or to learn about clinical trials.

American Cancer Society: www.cancer.org

National Institute of Health: www.nih.gov

Skin Cancer Foundation: www.skincancer.org

American College of Mohs Micrographic Surgery: www.mohscollege.org

www.clinicaltrials.gov

Melanoma Research Foundation: www.melanoma.org

www.melanomavaccine.com

American Academy of Dermatology: www.aad.org

www.ellenmarmur.com

8

Skin SOS: Problems and Prescriptions

think many people consider it a luxury to visit a dermatologist. Even those who suffer from chronic acne or psoriasis often don't seek help. Perhaps they believe it will go away on its own (it may not) or that it's not serious enough to see a doctor (it probably is). A skin condition can be a significant health problem and can negatively affect all aspects of a person's life. Another reason people avoid going is that many dermatologists do not take insurance and a lot of treatments that are considered cosmetic are not covered (such as removal of skin tags or the laser treatment of rosacea). It can be difficult and frustrating to navigate this system, but there are free clinics available and ways to get serious skin diseases treated. There's nothing that makes me as sad as being on the subway and seeing someone who's looking down at his or her feet, suffering and feeling ugly because he or she has cystic acne or a terrible rash—especially since, as a doctor, I know there are tools that will really help.

Some dermatologists concentrate primarily on antiaging cosmetic

procedures. But many dermatologists (like myself) treat a wide range
of conditions from cosmetic issues to skin cancer. In a single day, I will
biopsy a possible malignancy, perform a laser treatment on a patient's
brown spots, and attend to conditions like eczema, acne, or rosacea.
Doctors are problem solvers, and the following are common skin
issues that we treat all the time. Each is a brief snapshot: what I would
explain and advise for you if you were sitting in my office dealing with
the problem at hand. What is it, and why is it occurring? Is it dangerous? What can be done to resolve it? I can't recommend highly enough
the importance of visiting your own dermatologist if something on
your skin troubles you, hurts you, or even just annoys you. Most of
the time, there is a way to solve it, and there's no reason to suffer. To
get help finding a dermatologist, check www.aad.org.

It's important that your doctor emphasize the risks involved in any
kind of treatment. He or she should clearly explain the process to the
patient and encourage realistic expectations. Chemical peels and lasers
are not magic wands that sweep over your skin and fix something in
one easy step. These treatments can take longer than you think (and
cost more than you anticipated), there will probably be some pain, you
may need recovery time, and often there are side effects to consider.
Just as we shouldn't discount all skin conditions as superficial and cosmetic, we can't downplay the seriousness of the medical procedures
used to treat them. I hope this chapter will provide a helpful primer
and lay the groundwork to get you asking intelligent, thoughtful questions of your own physician. The issues in this chapter are organized
alphabetically, making it easy for you to flip to a particular problem
and find out how to fix it.

the problem: Acne

WHAT A DOCTOR CALLS IT: *Acne vulgaris*

WHAT IS IT?

There are two types of acne: comedonal (blackheads or whiteheads) and inflammatory (pimples). Dermatologists diagnose acne as mild, moderate, or severe. (Don't be alarmed if a dermatologist refers to your one or two zits as "acne." Doctors don't use the term "breakouts," so acne from our perspective doesn't necessarily mean chronically broken-out, oily skin.) Severe acne can consist of many papules (pimples) and deeper cysts (cystic acne).

WHY DOES IT HAPPEN?

Acne triggers can be hormonal changes (which is why so many teenagers and pregnant women suffer from it). Instigators also include genetics, certain foods (such as junk foods), and stress. Anything irritating that is put on your skin or done to it, intentionally or not (from a glycolic lotion to scrubbing too hard), can generate an inflammatory response that pops up as one pimple—or a few.

How does an acne pimple form in the first place? Going back to the anatomy lesson in chapter 1, the sebaceous gland is attached to a hair follicle. When that follicle is obstructed with dead keratinocytes, the oil doesn't have a way to get out. The *Proprionibacterium acnes* (*P. acnes*) bacteria that normally live harmoniously in the skin begin feasting on that glut of oil and give off toxic free fatty acids that perforate the base of the follicle, releasing toxins into the dermis. This sets off an immediate inflammatory response in the body and neutrophils (bacteria-fighting inflammatory cells) race to the area. The accumulation of these white neutrophils creates a pustule.

HOW CAN I PREVENT IT?

If you have acne-prone skin, take a good, hard look at your lifestyle, your stress level, what you put on your face every day, and what you are eating. Do some detective work on your particular triggers, and then try to avoid or adjust them. And be sure to choose the right ingredients in your cleanser, moisturizer, and sunscreen (see chapter 4 for the appropriate products for you).

Use products containing salicylic acid to keep the pores open and prevent obstruction, which starts the acne process in the first place. A prescription retinoid works beautifully to control both comedonal and inflammatory acne because it exfoliates the skin, regulates the shedding process of keratinocytes, and controls overproduction of sebum. For those with sensitive skin, I recommend using a retinoid three nights a week—applying it for fifteen minutes, then rinsing it off. These short treatments will be effective and less irritating. (Many patients find retinoids too harsh on their skin and then give up entirely.) The frequency and duration of retinoid applications may be increased once a tolerance has been established. The medication should be used until the skin clears, at which point the patient can taper off the applications.

HOW CAN I TREAT IT MYSELF?

Acne medication is a very big business, and that is a great thing, since drugstore aisles are filled with effective acne antidotes. Besides prescription retinoids and over-the-counter salicylic acid products that keep pores unplugged, sulfa medications (such as medicated pads and prescription cleansers) work to kill bacteria and calm inflammation. Benzoyl peroxide (in a concentration of 4% to 8%) is both an antibacterial and a keratolytic, so it dissolves the obstruction in the pore and kills off bacteria.

New at-home (over-the-counter) LED light gadgets claim to kill *P. acnes* bacteria with heat, like the light sources doctors use. These are far less powerful, but basically they microwave the bacteria. They do work, up to a point. If you have a more serious acne problem than one or two pimples, this method isn't going to be enough. It could be a great way to augment your treatment.

WHAT CAN A DOCTOR DO?

I urge anyone with moderate to severe acne not to go it alone. See a dermatologist who can help put together an individualized plan of attack. There's a world of medical options available to treat and control the condition, and there's no reason to suffer. Trying to treat acne yourself, even with the excellent OTC products out there, is frustrating and futile when the condition is serious. The gold standard of acne treatment is topical and systemic medications. We start with these, and if they don't provide the desired results, a doctor can offer other solutions, like chemical peels and laser treatments. A dermatologist who treats someone immediately with lasers or peels, without starting that patient on medications first, is not providing the best treatment for acne. Peels and lasers are a great addition to, and can accelerate the impact of medications but should be considered the primary prescription only if a patient cannot tolerate antibiotics, Accutane, or topical retinoic acid.

Here are the common courses of action that a dermatologist will use to treat acne. Every acne condition is as unique as the patient who suffers from it, so a skilled doctor will individualize the treatment— often combining a few of the following therapies—to achieve the best results with the fewest side effects.

PRESCRIPTION TOPICAL MEDICATIONS FOR ACNE

As I mentioned, a prescription retinoid keeps acne in control by regulating cell turnover and keeping the pores unblocked, which is half the battle. Sulfa medications, benzoyl peroxide, and antibiotic cleansers— all in prescription strength—are effective too. Topical antibiotics such as clindamycin are anti-inflammatory and antibacterial, so they calm redness and kill *P. acnes.*

Most people don't want to use a bunch of different lotions, gels, and liquids if they can just use one. (In a compliance study, researchers placed a computer chip inside the cap of a medication container to record every time it was opened. Though most patients said they applied the cream twice a day as prescribed, the computer chip proved that they hardly opened the tube.) The newest acne products—for example, a prescription cleanser that contains both benzoyl peroxide and clindamycin—multitask and make it easier for patients to be compliant with at-home treatment. There's now a prescription acne gel that combines an antibiotic with a retinoid, a one-two punch that's especially successful in treating adult-onset acne.

Usually a patient with severe acne takes one oral medication once or twice a day, applies a topical retinoid at night, and uses one topical benzoyl peroxide antibiotic (such as BenzaClin wash). It's a lot to remember and a long process to endure, but the results are worth the effort.

SYSTEMIC MEDICATIONS FOR ACNE

Acne patients take antibiotics and a vitamin A derivative orally, as well as applying them topically, so they work from the inside out too. Antibiotics are used for inflammatory acne and isotretinoin (a vitamin A analog known by the brand name Accutane) for both comedonal and inflammatory forms.

Antibiotics like tetracycline are prescribed in an eight-week course, usually in conjunction with a topical retinoid and a benzoyl peroxide–antibiotic cleanser. These days doctors are gravitating more to a new generation of low-dose antibiotics that have fewer side effects and will hopefully prevent antibiotic resistance. (Higher-dose antibiotics have been known to cause gastrointestinal problems and yeast infections.) These medications, such as Doryx, Solodyn, and Oracea, aren't as harsh and have a similar, positive anti-inflammatory effect—but they have little if no antibacterial strength. Another excellent medicine is spironolactone. Originally a diuretic, its anti-testosterone effects diminish acne—especially the persistent acne around the mouth.

If oral antibiotics fail, isotretinoin (Accutane) is the next step.

There are many options to try before this is prescribed, since Accutane is the biggest gun you can use against acne. It's a very serious solution, but I feel that Accutane is a miracle drug. It's a systemic retinoid that works in the same way the topical medication does (by regulating cell turnover and decreasing oil production), but it is much stronger. It's the only thing that works for certain patients and is incredibly successful in most cases. Usually patients take a four-month course of the drug. It is often prescribed in conjunction with topical medications, such as benzoyl peroxide washes. There is a significant risk of a flare-up of acne once Accutane is started, and if that happens your doctor can prescribe systemic antibiotics or steroids to calm it down. Within two months patients usually see a good improvement in their skin.

Some people taking Accutane have suffered side effects such as headaches, depression, paranoia and (rarely) even suicidal tendencies. There is also a significant risk of birth defects, so female patients must be on birth control during treatment with Accutane. More commonly, the side effects are photosensitivity, bone pain, dry skin (even dry eyes and lips), and hair loss. These are often dose-related (and reversible). Dosage depends on the weight of the patient, usually ranging between 10 and 60 milligrams per day. The drug stays in the system for at least one hundred days after the patient takes the last dose, which is important for pregnancy issues and for any surgical procedures (the drug interferes with wound healing). Though there's much ambivalence about it, I believe that the drug is safe to take under a doctor's supervision, given that it is under strict regulation and restrictions by the FDA. (Both doctors and patients must join a national registry called iPLEDGE before prescribing or taking the drug.) Admittedly, this sounds like quite an involved process to get an acne prescription. Perhaps because of this, there has been a disturbing trend among young women to purchase the medication online. Self-prescription and buying pills from who knows where can be extremely unsafe. Please understand that this is a very serious medication with very real side effects, which must be administered and monitored by a physician.

MEDICAL PROCEDURES FOR ACNE

Again, acne is a complex condition and every single case is different, so it's difficult to describe a general treatment. I have to look at a patient's skin in order to diagnose and treat it properly. Some patients can't tolerate oral medications or have sensitive skin that simply can't handle topical retinoids. Some try these things and still need more help. I frequently utilize one of the following treatments to enhance or hasten the effects of gold-standard medications.

LASER AND LIGHT TREATMENTS FOR ACNE

A v-beam laser (which is actually made to target blood vessels) and intense pulsed light treatments both act by killing off *P. acnes* bacteria, shrinking the sebaceous glands and reducing the number of inflammatory neutrophils in the follicle. It may even be that the liquid nitrogen spray on some lasers, used as a cooling mechanism, might kill off *P. acnes* in the follicle.

The same photodynamic therapy (PDT) used to treat pre–skin cancers can be effective in killing *P. acnes* bacteria and treating inflammatory acne. Aminolevulinic acid (ALA) is applied to the skin and is absorbed by the bacteria. Then a special blue light (multiple BLU-U) activates the acid and causes a chemical reaction that destroys the illuminated bacteria and shrinks oil glands.

From a patient advocate standpoint, it's important to know that many doctors have only one laser. So they have no choice but to use it, whether or not it's the most effective one for the job at hand. Before getting any laser treatment, look at the laser chart (in chapter 10, pages 332–333), which explains each laser and its specific function. Some lasers, like the Vbeam are meant to affect blood vessels, while Fraxel is best for resurfacing and deep exfoliation. With this basic know-how, you can pose detailed, researched questions to your doctor, such as: What about trying PDT, or is a chemical peel better for treating this? Will IPL work as well as a laser, or will it take many more treatments to see improvement?

CHEMICAL PEELS FOR ACNE

I have used a combination of 30% TCA chemical peels and laser treatments on teenagers with severe comedonal or pustular (inflammatory) acne, and now they have calm, beautiful skin. A peel followed by microdermabrasion works wonders for patients who cannot tolerate Accutane. (Again, every acne condition is unique, and I tailor a combination of therapies to each individual patient's condition.) It's important to stop all medication three days before a peel or PDT and three days afterward. A peel stings and burns a lot for about twenty minutes during the treatment. The patient's skin is pink for the first three days, then becomes dry and begins to peel. Usually by day 10 the skin is much improved. The most important advice: don't pick your skin. It is so tempting while it's peeling, but this can harm your skin since the pieces are still attached. When the skin is dry, using a noncomedogenic, fragrance-free moisturizer can help soften the skin and reduce the temptation to pick. You can use a wet, soapy washcloth to gently massage your face in circular motions to slough off the dead skin.

CORTISONE INJECTIONS FOR PIMPLES

An injection of hydrocortisone, an anti-inflammatory steroid, is a good quick fix for eradicating an acne bump—but not a practical solution when there are many pimples. (Injecting multiple papules on a regular basis could lead to pitted acne scars later, since a risk of cortisone is atrophy.) The injection itself releases some of the pressure, and the cortisone acts as an anti-inflammatory so it turns off the neutrophils and flattens the papule. It's especially helpful for people who tend to make scars, as it avoids massive demolition of the dermis by toxic free fatty acids. The perfect type of pimple to inject is a red, painful cyst that hasn't come up yet because the cortisone nips it in the bud and stops the demolition from occurring. The pimple usually goes away in twelve to twenty-four hours.

New (and sometimes pricey) treatments are always entering the acne-fighting market. The latest is a new technology that uses micro-dermabrasion to exfoliate and unplug the pores followed by a light treatment to kill *P. acnes* bacteria. It's getting tons of press, supposedly requires very little to no downtime, and is meant to work on mild to moderate acne cases. Essentially this new method utilizes preexisting technologies that are well tolerated, and it should be a good way to improve acne. Your doctor should always direct you to the gold standard solution first, however: topical and oral medications. The cosmetic treatments that I know work (and that I use in my office), either in conjunction with or instead of these medications, are lasers and chemical peels.

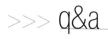 >>> q&a

Q: Why am I breaking out in zits when I have extremely dry skin? Is this acne?

A: No, it's more like an acne imposter and shouldn't be treated in the same way you would acne (i.e., by drying out pimples and killing bacteria with benzoyl peroxide). What you have is an "acneiform" reaction pattern that mimics acne. There are tiny papules filled with neutrophils, but there are no *P. acnes* bacteria, nor is there keratin plugging the pore. It's an inflammatory response to a stress on the skin—in your case dehydration. Seasonal changes and environmental variations can cause them too, which is why you may break out in these pimples on vacation. Some people get these breakouts as a reaction to waxing or bleaching facial hair or from an irritating ingredient in a skin care product—even simple soap. Therefore, using harsh acne medications to dry out the pimples is the wrong tactic and will make the problem even worse. If you moisturize your skin to counteract the dryness, the inflammatory papules will go away.

Q: What is adult-onset acne, and why do I have to deal with it? I feel like a pre-pubescent teen, but I'm in my forties. Should I use antiaging products or acne medications?

A: Having acne as an adult is truly frustrating and puzzling. The prime trigger is similar to that of teenage acne, namely hormonal changes. Other factors come into play too, of course, such as diet, stress, and the wrong skin care products. Adult-onset acne tends to be perioral, distributed around the mouth. I prescribe benzoyl peroxide to clear up the pimples and a topical retinoid to regulate keratinocytes and keep the pores clear. Often a systemic solution is necessary to get rid of tenacious acne. A doctor may prescribe a low-dose antibiotic or a medication called spironolactone or Aldactone, which has antitestosterone properties that reduce oil production in the skin.

Women may find that pimples pop up more just before their periods, when androgen hormones such as testosterone stimulate the sebaceous glands to pump out more oil. You tend to break out when testosterone levels peak. I always ask my female patients who complain of acne if their periods are normal and if they have any hormonal issues. Menopause can be a trigger, and so can polycystic ovarian syndrome (PCOS). Adult acne can be a symptom of PCOS, and I've often made that diagnosis by looking at a woman's skin. Hormone therapy, usually in the form of birth control pills, can help regulate testosterone and estrogen levels, keeping them on a more even keel. Though some brands of birth control pills have sought FDA approval specifically for antiacne claims, all combination contraceptive pills (those that contain both estrogen and progestin) work in the same way to fight acne: by maintaining hormone stability.

It's important to make sure that what you think is acne is not an inflammatory response to irritation or rosacea. There's an overlap between these conditions because the pimples generated by both mimic acne, but their treatment differs greatly. If a woman in her fifties or sixties has acne, I suspect it may actually be rosacea, which tends to worsen over the course of your life since it's exacerbated by sun damage.

Q: What's the deal with Proactiv Solution? Do the products really work, and why?

A: Sold originally through infomercials, Proactiv Solution has become the best-selling acne line in the world. The two dermatologists who developed it understood the psychology of compliance and its importance to successful acne treatment. They didn't invent any new medications per se but came up with an at-home skin care system that's easy to use. It's similar to a diet system like The Zone, in which prepared meals are ready and waiting for you—so following the plan is a no-brainer. The system works by simplifying treatment for mild to moderate acne and utilizing effective, traditional ingredients (primarily benzoyl peroxide and sulfur).

It's important to note that products with higher concentrations of benzoyl peroxide can dry out and also bleach skin (and linens and towels that come into contact with it). Some people wonder why the products seem to stop working after a while. The problem is with the acne, not with the skin care system. The benzoyl peroxide in Proactiv Solution and other over-the-counter acne products kills P. acnes bacteria, but often the bacteria become resistant to the medication. For this reason, you have to keep changing your mode of attack. This is one reason why acne is such a big business: each person's acne changes, and treatments have to be rotated accordingly—almost to keep the acne bacteria guessing.

Q: Does acne in someone with darker skin have to be treated differently.

A: Dark skin has a slightly different healing process and tends to be more sensitive when it comes to acne, so it can be more difficult to treat. This type of skin is more prone to developing dark marks (postinflammatory hyperpigmentation) from pimples and from topical acne medications like benzoyl peroxide. Consequently, oral acne medications such as antibiotics or Accutane work better for patients whose dark skin tends to pigment easily. Postinflammatory hyperpigmentation (PIH) will gradually fade over time. To accelerate the process, a light chemical peel (one with glycolic acid, which is gentler on sensitive skin) exfoliates the scarring from the skin. Combination therapy with acne medication and lasers is another good option. More than ever, you need to have an experienced doctor do your laser treatments (since this too can cause PIH), and I recommend, before having laser done on your face, having small test spots done first to make sure that your skin is compatible with the laser technology.

Q: Is it really so bad to pop a zit? Doesn't the pore need to be open for any medication to get in and work? And does toothpaste or eye drops really work to get rid of a pimple?

A: I know it's tempting, but popping a pimple can lead to infection and end up creating a scar. Believe me, benzoyl peroxide will get in there, dry out those anti-inflammatory neutrophils, and clear it up without your popping it first. Like salicylic acid, it disintegrates the top layer of skin. Using pressure to pop a zit pushes bacteria and free fatty acids back inside the skin. Think of the follicle as being like a tiny balloon filled with toxic material that's going to pop internally—that's when scarring happens.

As for toothpaste, it's not my first choice, but I think it can work by essentially desiccating the area with astringents. Many pastes also contain silica, which is a drying agent. Be careful of using toothpastes with fluoride or menthol, which are highly irritating to the skin and can cause more pimples as an inflammatory response. Eye drops that claim to "get the red out" of eyes are said to do the same for an inflamed pimple. (Models and makeup artists have been using this trick on photo shoots for years.) The ingredient in the drops, tetrahydrozaline hydrochloride, is a vasoconstrictor, so it might reduce skin redness too. But it's certainly not going to eradicate the bacteria and oil that form the papule. Bottom line: if you're desperate, on a desert

A

island with no benzoyl peroxide in sight, and only some toothpaste and eye drops, give it a try—but don't expect a miracle. (Although I confess that I do use toothpaste on a pimple if I'm desperate when I'm traveling.)

the problem: Acne Scars

WHAT IS IT?

Like most scars, the byproducts of acne are generated by trauma to the skin that leads to abnormal collagen formation. Just imagine how much trauma the epidermis and the dermis goes through with acne: all that bacteria and those toxic free fatty acids destroy collagen, and the new collagen being made to replace it is produced hastily. This results in some shoddy construction, forming bulky raised scars and bumps, and pitted indentations.

Those open indentations are called patulous or atrophic scars, and there are ice pick scars that look like tiny indented slivers on the skin. Hypertrophic scars are raised and sometimes red, keloid scars are even larger bulky bumps of abnormal tissue. Papular scars are white bumps, and they are difficult to get rid of. And there are brown spots, or post-inflammatory hyperpigmentation, which is common in darker skin.

WHY DOES IT HAPPEN, AND HOW CAN I PREVENT IT?

One of our goals in medical acne treatment is to prevent scarring, but the inflammation and trauma generated by acne often leave scars behind. Don't make them worse by overusing products that will irritate the skin. Stick with tried-and-true benzoyl peroxide and salicylic acid, but don't pile on other acids or harsh ingredients such as menthol on top of it. Don't pick at your acne, and don't pop pimples. Self-acne surgery pushes bacteria and free fatty acids back into the skin and is a sure way to create a scar.

A

WHAT CAN A DOCTOR DO?

If your acne is pretty much gone and you have brown spots left, a program of sunscreen, prescription retinoids, and bleaching creams will help diminish the hyperpigmentation. Retinoids can also increase collagen growth, which can eventually improve the look of pitted scars and smooth the overall texture of the skin. A chemical peel or Fraxel laser resurfacing can hasten the process even more.

Dermabrasion is another procedure that works well for all scars by sculpting a raised mark flat using electrocautery, mechanical dermabrasion, or a resurfacing laser such as CO_2 or erbium: YAG (see "The Problem: A Scar" on page 236). Larger hypertrophic and keloid scars can be injected with hydrocortisone to shrink the bulk of the collagen and flatten the scar.

For indented scars—patulous or atrophic scars and ice-pick scars—there are a few fairly extreme options. I must underscore that there's no magic wand for acne scars, and improving their appearance is the goal. It's important to realize that this is an improvement, not perfection.

I prefer using a fractionated laser (such as Fraxel) to thermally fill in inverted acne scars by building collagen over a span of six months. I've had great results, but it's a matter of economics for some people, since the treatment is expensive and can require up to ten sessions. (The price could end up being close to $15,000.)

Another alternative for patulous and ice-pick scars is injecting hyaluronic acid filler into the area. This decreases the shadow effect by plumping up the indentation and providing a more even texture. It provides immediate gratification, whereas Fraxel takes time to produce collagen. (I like to use both methods together.) The problem is that this is a temporary filler that will be resorbed into the skin after about a year, so the procedure will have to be repeated. For those who don't want to get annual injections of filler or can't afford Fraxel, acne surgery is an excellent option. The scar tissue is excised and the two healthy edges of skin are pulled together with a stitch. The patient is left with some tiny scars, but they are almost imperceptible.

the problem: Blackheads, Whiteheads, and Milia

WHAT A DOCTOR CALLS THEM: comedones (an open comedone is a blackhead; a closed comedone is a whitehead)

WHAT ARE THEY?

Comedones (blackheads and whiteheads) are how dermatologists refer to bumps or little cysts on the skin caused by a blockage of pores or hair follicles. They are forms of acne and can frequently be accompanied by pimples elsewhere on the skin. Like acne, a blackhead, or open comedone, is formed when dead keratinocytes block the pore, oxidize in the open air, and turn black. It is *not* dirt! The oxidized keratin on top is black, but underneath it's white.

Because a closed comedone is covered by the epidermis, the cyst remains white. In fact, although it appears to be right under the surface of the skin, a whitehead is actually in the dermis, so trying to extract one will cause trauma to the skin. Whiteheads and milia are very similar—both are closed-over keratin plugs—but milia are not associated with acne. They are caused by aging and slower cell turnover. Milia are tiny white bumps formed by trapped keratin compacted in the pore, but there is no bacteria or oil involved.

WHY DO THEY HAPPEN?

Both open and closed comedones form in the same way that acne does: a buildup of sebum and dead skin cells clogs the inside of a pore and forms a small cyst. Both blackheads and whiteheads can become infected with the same bacteria that cause acne. Milia, however, is a case of keratin-obstructed pores caused by skin that isn't shedding normally. It is not an acne issue and happens frequently as we age; it generally starts to show up in your thirties. Milia can also be a side effect of laser resurfacing, because the skin is growing at an accelerated

B

rate (as a wound-healing response) and can trap keratin inside the pores.

HOW CAN I PREVENT THEM?

All three of these pore-blocking problems can be kept in check with regular exfoliation and the use of retinoids, which not only slough off dead skin cells but regulate the shedding process. A chemical exfoliant (salicylic or glycolic acid) or a mechanical method (such as a scrub or at-home microdermabrasion) can be used once or twice a week. If the problem is chronic, see a dermatologist for microdermabrasion or chemical peels twice a year. (I like to do it when the seasons change, the winter to spring transition and then summer to fall. Skin tends to be thicker and duller due to the environmental exposure of the winter and summer, and more in need of professional exfoliation.)

HOW CAN I TREAT THEM MYSELF?

Treat comedones with salicylic acid to keep pores open and prescription retinoids to regulate keratinocytes. My best prescription is augmenting topical retinoids with regular exfoliation. As with acne, prevention and at-home treatment go hand in hand. Since people with dry skin seem to make more milia, be sure to moisturize after exfoliating or using a retinoid product.

WHAT CAN A DOCTOR DO?

Besides prescribing a retinoid medication, a dermatologist can consider putting a patient on Accutane if a comedonal acne problem is extreme. I've found that another effective remedy is a 20% or 30% TCA chemical peel, followed a week later by microdermabrasion to slough off the dead, peeling skin. After this process I manually extract any comedones that are left over. Usually three peels a year can keep the condition under control. Fractionated laser works well too, by literally drilling microscopic holes into the surface of the skin and into the cysts to release the trapped keratin. Microdermabrasion alone is incredibly effective for treating comedones and milia. Generally, people have microdermabrasion once a week for two or three months.

If retinoic acid and exfoliation aren't working to control milia, a dermatologist can extract them. First the area is numbed with a topical anesthetic; then the doctor pierces the top of the cyst with a needle and extracts the keratin with a comedone extractor, a tiny bowl with a hole in the bottom. The doctor presses the convex side of the surface over the comedone, and the keratin is released. Another option is burning the top using electrocautery, then extracting larger cysts and letting the smaller milia slough off by themselves. If there are multiple milia to extract (which is often the case), a chemical peel will strip off the top layer of skin and get rid of them in one fell swoop. (Because a peel isn't as deep as laser resurfacing, it usually won't end up generating more milia as the skin renews itself.) All of these methods are fairly painful and require four to eight days of recovery time; even more unfortunately, milia will slowly accumulate again. Regular exfoliation should impede that process.

>>> skin lie: Tiny white bumps under the eyes are caused by heavy skin cream that clogs the pores.

>>> skin truth: Those tiny white spots can be due to plenty of things (all genetic), but using rich moisturizing cream isn't one of them. They may be milia or even seborrheic kerotoses, which sometimes show up as tiny, smooth bumps, not scaly lesions. (See the explanation of seborrheic keratosis on page 238.) Some people get skin tags (discussed later on page 239) under their eyes. Another possibility might be syringomas, benign sweat duct cysts that are often clustered on the eyelids and under the eyes. The loss of elastin (thanks to aging and sun damage) can create a condition called solar elastosis, in which the thin skin under the eyes sinks down onto the remaining collagen and looks bumpy, with a texture like an orange peel.

Those with darker skin often get smooth, brown bumps as well. These genetic bumps, called dermatosis papulosis nigrans, are benign and show up under the eyes and upper cheeks and sometimes over the nose. There's no reason to worry about them, but if they bother you aesthetically they can be removed with electrocautery (although new ones will eventually take their place).

the problem: Brown Spots

WHAT A DOCTOR CALLS THEM: solar lentigines

WHAT IS IT?

Questions about dark discoloration and brown spots (and how to remove them) are definitely the most frequently asked by patients, the press, and my friends. Hyperpigmentation is an overproduction of melanin in a certain area, as a response to UV exposure. Hypopigmentation is another sign of sun damage that results in white spots, like confetti sprinkled on the skin. This happens when the sun basically fries the melanocytes in that area and they can no longer produce pigment at all—leaving those spots especially vulnerable to sun damage.

WHY DO THEY HAPPEN?

These spots are dubbed "sun spots" for a good reason: they are caused exclusively by sun damage. Melanocytes have produced excess melanin in some spots in an effort to protect the skin from UV rays.

HOW CAN I PREVENT THEM?

Wear sunscreen every single day and stay out of the sun whenever possible.

HOW CAN I TREAT THEM MYSELF?

Topical lightening agents such as kojic acid and hydroquinone will fade brown spots over time, but that can require a long wait. Spot treatments with over-the-counter-strength kojic acid and 2% hydroquinone can take at least six months to work, since they are so mild.

Someone with even moderate hyperpigmentation should see a dermatologist not only to take care of the problem (with prescription-strength medication or cosmetic procedures) but to make sure that any discoloration is *not* skin cancer. A new patient recently came to me about removing a dark spot on his temple. It was his only brown mark, and I biopsied it. It turned out to be melanoma. This is an increasingly common occurrence in my practice. Obviously, it's a smart idea to have a doctor take a look at any brown spots for health reasons, then minister to them cosmetically.

WHAT CAN A DOCTOR DO?

Topical hydroquinone, a derivative of benzene, doesn't literally bleach the skin but suppresses overactive melanocytes and slows down the pigment-making process. Hydroquinone alone is applied directly onto the dark spot and slowly erases it within at least six months (although it could be sooner). It works by blocking the enzyme tyrosinase inside the melanocytes that makes melanin. A doctor's prescription increases the concentration from 2% (what you get OTC) to 4% or 6%, but beyond that is unsafe. In fact, the FDA proposed a ban on over-the-counter sales of hydroquinone in 2006 because too strong a dose or using even a lower dose for an extended period of time causes side effects such as darkening and thickening of the skin (exogenous ochronosis). The chemical has also been shown to act as a carcinogen in mice. Other topical treatments combine hydroquinone with a retinoid and a light anti-inflammatory steroid. Another uses hydroquinone with glycolic acid to lighten and exfoliate the skin.

Lasers that target pigment, such as the Ruby and the Q-switched ND:YAG, work better than more surface-level treatments like chemical peels, microdermabrasion, or intense pulsed light (IPL) treatments. A laser can reach melanosomes deep in the skin and might even be able to get rid of a brown spot in one treatment (although two or three treatments may be necessary to do the trick). I use topical medications and laser treatments together, but many people haven't had success with hydroquinone or don't want to use it, so lasers alone can be very effective. Laser light converts to heat and blows up the melanosomes, after which they flake off the skin. (It feels like a hot snap against your skin but lasts only a few seconds; then it stings for a few minutes right afterward.) Strangely enough, darker spots go away faster than lighter ones because there is more pigment for the laser to aim for; a pale spot is an almost invisible target. The procedure takes just a few minutes (and, as always, numbing cream is applied to the skin first), but the downtime is up to a week. The skin will get red and then scab, so recovery time takes at least five days. (From the neck down it could be anywhere from two to four weeks because the skin there is thicker and slower to heal.)

the problem: A Bruise

WHAT A DOCTOR CALLS IT: ecchymosis

WHAT IS IT?

A bruise is blood that has extravasated (or migrated) outside the blood vessel because of trauma. Tiny blood vessels near the surface of the skin can burst from a bump, a scrape, or injection—any kind of physical distress. Bruises change color like a mood ring as they mature (from black and blue to green to yellow) and last about one week on the face and two weeks on the body.

WHY DOES IT HAPPEN, AND HOW CAN I PREVENT IT?

Most people don't remember bumping themselves and panic when they find a big bruise. Some people actually scratch their skin during sleep and wake up with purple streaks, not knowing where they came from. If you bruise easily, it's likely that you are taking some kind of medication that thins the blood. Many of us take aspirin or ibuprofen, which acts as a blood thinner. Prescription medications such as clopidogrel bisulfate (Plavix), taken for heart conditions, do the same and increase the risk of bruising and bleeding. Even supplements such as omega-3 fatty acids, vitamin E, St. John's wort, and ginkgo biloba thin the blood, as does eating a lot of garlic. Raise the issue with your doctor if you seem to be bruising more than normal. You may need blood tests to rule out a genetic bleeding disorder, or you may need to adjust your medication.

HOW CAN I TREAT IT MYSELF?

There's not much you can do for a simple bruise. *Arnica montana* is a homeopathic medication (available at health food stores) that claims to make bruises fade away faster. Many of my patients swear by it. You can apply a topical cream or tincture to the skin, take homeopathic pills, or both.

WHAT CAN A DOCTOR DO?

Usually, a bruise doesn't necessitate a visit to the doctor. But if it becomes very swollen or more painful than bruises you've had in the past, or if you can feel firmness under the skin, it should be checked. Sometimes bruising can cause a hematoma, which happens when a lot of blood seeps out from the vessel and then coagulates like jelly. This collection of blood can go so far as to organize itself into a hard clot the consistency of wood. Both of these are very dangerous and usually occur after there's been major trauma (such as a surgical procedure) to the area. Left unattended, this congealed blood can lead to a devastating bacterial infection. A clot can break into chunks, migrate to somewhere else in the body, and block a vessel, causing a heart attack or a stroke. To treat a hematoma, a doctor must open up the skin surgically and expel the congealed mass or the clot. It's a painful, but vital, outpatient procedure.

the problem: A Callus

WHAT IS IT?
A callus is a form of hyperkeratosis, or thickened skin, that creates a hard surface.

WHY DOES IT HAPPEN?
A callus can develop on any area of skin that is repeatedly exposed to friction or pressure. As a reaction to this constant contact, layers of dead skin form to protect and cushion the vulnerable spot. Runners and dancers often get calluses on their heels or the balls of their feet (and wearing uncomfortable or too-tight shoes causes them too, as most women know). Weight lifters, tennis players, and construction workers form this tough skin on their palms. I have one on the inside of my thumb from playing squash. A callus can even show up on the outside of the ankle if a person always sits with that foot crossed over the other knee and tends to move the foot back and forth nervously.

HOW CAN I PREVENT IT?
It's simple: identify the action that may be causing the callus, and stop it. Or let it be, since it is providing a cushion over bones, nerves, and tendons. If you have a callus somewhere on the foot, try switching your shoes everyday so you don't always put pressure on the same area.

HOW CAN I TREAT IT MYSELF?
Moisturize the callused area twice a day with a thick cream containing either urea (Carmol lotion) or lactic acid (AmLactin or Lac-Hydrin), both of which have exfoliating and humectant properties. This will help to thin and soften the skin buildup, making it easier to exfoliate the top layers with a pumice stone. If you use an abrasive tool, such as pumice, to slough off the callus, be gentle. Aggressive scrubbing can worsen the situation—remember why the callus formed in the first place (friction and pressure).

WHAT CAN A DOCTOR DO?

A callus is usually not dangerous or painful. If it does begin to hurt, it may be overlying a nerve, or it may be a sign of an anatomical problem. For example, people with bunions on their feet usually form deposits of dead tissue there to cushion the protruding bone at the edge of the foot near the big toe. Hence, the callus is covering and padding the real problem. In a case like this, I advise seeing a podiatrist or an orthopedic surgeon. A dermatologist can pare down the top layers of a callus with a surgical blade, but it will return if the same action or friction on the area is repeated or if an underlying medical problem remains. I would trust a doctor, but not a nail technician, to perform this simple procedure, and don't try it yourself since it's easy to cut too far and hit living tissue.

>>> q&a
_____

Q: Is there anything I can do to get rid of cellulite?

A: It's pretty unanimous that we all hate our cellulite, so I suppose if there were a remedy that worked, most of us would pay anything for it. There wouldn't be a debate, just a waiting list. Sadly, there is no real cure yet.

Cellulite is caused less by the amount of fat present than by the structure of the fat and skin together. Fibrous anchors go from the epidermis down to the fat layer, and those little connections cause the dimpling appearance. Cellulite is genetic and doesn't mean you are fat. Even people who are in awesome shape can have cellulite. Many young, gorgeous, and fit women have cellulite. Exercise and a healthy diet can improve the problem by reducing fat but probably won't eliminate it completely.

Liposuction is the most effective treatment to improve the puckering appearance, but since it's impossible to change the architecture of the skin, it's not the perfect answer. The fat that is left will probably start dimpling again. There is also a risk of uneven distribution of the remaining fat and of indentations. Once a young woman, an athlete, came to my office after having a liposuction treatment on her thighs that had left an indentation the size of a plum. I used injectable filler to normalize the dented area. Cellulite treatments such as Endermologie (using a massaging device with rollers and a suction hose) or meso-therapy (involving injections of botanicals, vitamins, and minerals to break up the fat cells) claim to reduce cellulite. In my opinion, they don't. They can't disintegrate fat or disconnect the anchors that are causing cellulite, and neither can the slew of "firming" cellulite creams and gels. As with most topicals, any visible results wash off or fade away fast. Again, if any one of these really worked, it would be the hot-test product on the market.

The newest cellulite-fighting procedures use a low-energy laser plus massage or radio frequency, infrared light, and massage to reduce cellulite and smooth the appearance of the skin. These try to shrink the fat by heating it and liquefying it. For some people they may work somewhat, but both are far from home runs. They probably provide the short-term illusion of improvement because they cause swelling in the area that fills up the dimpling. You have to have a series of expen-sive treatments to see any results at all. Usually a patient has to have at least eight to fifteen sessions, and the results have been shown to last only a few months. Cellulite subscission is a new surgical technique that employs a needle to sever the anchors under the skin. This proce-dure, which is based on a successful treatment for acne scars, makes theoretical sense, although safety studies in the United States aren't plentiful and the surgery is expensive. My advice: save your money, let the cellulite battle go, and buy yourself a beautiful pair of shoes. That will have a much better payoff.

>>> skin lie: Dandruff is caused by dry skin.

>>> skin truth: Dandruff is usually due to a rash called seborrheic dermatitis, which can present as a flaky scalp. (Seborrheic dermatitis also shows up as itchy, flaky skin inside the ear, around the eyebrows, or in the nasal creases.) In some cases, dandruff is an inflammatory reaction to a yeast on the skin. Dandruff can also accompany psoriasis or a fungal infection of the scalp called tinea capitis (which occurs in children and teenagers). In each case, an inflammatory disorder causes accelerated cell turnover, which sets off the exfoliation and flaking. If you have chronic dandruff, see a dermatologist to be sure which condition is causing it. But the skin isn't flaking off because the scalp is dry. In fact, the best way to prevent dandruff is by washing your hair often, three or four times per week. This keeps the scalp clean and exfoliates dead skin from the surface. There are special dandruff shampoos that contain either selenium (which supposedly helps the exfoliation process) or pyrithione zinc (which kills off yeast). However, I'm not completely sold that these work any better than regular shampoo to get rid of dandruff. To treat seborrheic dermatitis on the scalp, a dermatologist prescribes a topical steroid foam medication to be used on a regular basis. The mousse formulation penetrates to the scalp quickly and acts as an anti-inflammatory. Because chronic use of topical steroids can be dangerous (causing thinning of the skin and possibly side effects to the endocrine system), new nonsteroidal medications are being formulated that may soon take their place.

D

the problem: Dark Circles under the Eyes

WHAT A DOCTOR CALLS THEM: infraorbital hyperpigmentation (although this refers to just one cause of the problem, pigmented skin)

WHAT ARE THEY, AND WHY DO THEY HAPPEN?

There are six explanations for dark circles, and accurately diagnosing which one is your particular issue will be key to finding a remedy. One is infraorbital hyperpigmentation, darkness concentrated on this area of skin, which is a genetic trait. To find out if that's your problem, gently pull the skin away from the hollow under the eye, making the area flat, which physically eliminates any shadow effect. If the darkness is still there, it's pigmented skin. Or two, you may have thin skin (due to either heredity or decreased collagen from aging) resting on dark muscle and blood vessels, which creates that dark semicircle under the eyes. Three, sometimes the circles are due to tiny blood vessels under the surface of the skin, another genetic feature. Four, you may have deeply inset bone structure, which produces a shadow from your brow bone to darken the area under the eye. Five, as we age the cheek and orbital bones dissolve, creating more of a shadow. And six, bruises after plastic surgery such as rhinoplasty (nose job) or blepharoplasty (eyelid surgery) can leave a rust-colored stain under the eyes called hemosiderin.

HOW CAN I PREVENT THEM?

Unfortunately, there's little one can do about a hereditary trait such as pigmented skin or the anatomical reality of thin skin under the eyes. Once they show up, dark circles can either be camouflaged with makeup or treated by a dermatologist. Dark circles can show up when you're exhausted too, because the parasympathetic system hasn't been able to drain and circulate fluid—including blood—properly during sleep. The result is venous congestion of the veins under the eyes

HOW CAN I TREAT THEM MYSELF?

Like over-the-counter antidotes for puffy eyes, the plethora of topical eye gels, serums, and creams probably isn't going to do much but moisturize (which isn't a bad thing; they just won't get rid of dark circles). Most contain kojic acid, a mild skin-lightening agent (which won't do anything if your circles aren't a hyperpigmentation problem). Some include vitamin K, which *inside* the body affects the clotting of the blood. Applied topically, it's supposed to diminish bruising and darkness associated with blood vessels. There is no research to support these claims, and, like many ingredients, it's unlikely to penetrate far enough into the dermis to affect blood vessels in a long-lasting way.

WHAT CAN A DOCTOR DO?

There are as many medical solutions as there are reasons for dark circles, and each is specific to the cause. If the issue is thinner skin resting over muscle, an injectable filler of either fat (taken from the patient's own supply somewhere else in the body) or hyaluronic acid (such as Restylane or Juvéderm) can change the optics and shape of the under-eye area. The translucent skin will now rest on yellow or clear filler above the muscle. The procedure also plumps up the infraorbital hollow, eliminating the shadow effect that lends a tired, droopy basset hound look to the face. Hyaluronic acid filler has also been shown to initiate collagen production where it's been injected. Temporary filler (fat and silicone are the only ones that are more permanent) usually needs to be reinjected every six to twelve months, although for many people it lasts a couple of years.

If the problem is prominent veins or hemosiderin near the eyes, a vascular beam laser will get rid of them. The treatment takes about ten minutes, but the patient may have to return at some point to repeat the treatment if new blood vessels regrow there in the next five to ten years. Three to five laser treatments are usually required.

Hyperpigmented skin is receptive to lasers, peels, and prescription topical creams such as hydroquinone. (In general, the same procedure a doctor would do for dark spots would be utilized for dark pigmentation under the eyes.) I use three methods of high-tech exfoliation: a fractionated laser (such as Fraxel), intense pulsed light (IPL) treatments that disintegrate pigment with heat, or chemical peels that lift the pigment off. (Ruby or YAG lasers that target pigment can be too strong to use on this delicate area.) IPL is not a true laser (it gives off multiple wavelengths, or a spectrum, of light rather than one laser beam), and it's not as specialized as a laser so it may take three times as many IPL treatments to get a successful effect. But the downtime for IPL is zero, which is why it's been tagged "the lunchtime laser." A fractionated laser can reduce the appearance of pigmented skin under the eyes by 50 to 80 percent. For most laser treatments (with the exception of Fraxel and IPL), the patient's eyeballs are numbed with drops and metal eye shields are placed over them to protect them from the laser's light (this is not as scary as it sounds, I promise!). Each of these laser treatments takes ten to thirty minutes and must be repeated four to eight times before improvement is apparent.

Certainly, using a prescription topical cream to fade the pigmentation over time sounds much easier, but it's hardly a quick fix or a sure thing. It takes a minimum of six weeks to see improvement, and if there is no change in six months you should stop using the medication. Hydroquinone, a skin-lightening cream, can be effective, but be careful to use the dosage prescribed by your doctor—a high percentage of hydroquinone can cause ochronosis, an even darker discoloration of the skin. Retinoids have been found to be helpful for hyperpigmentation because they slow down melanin production. Many dermatologists use a cream that contains a light steroid, a retinoid, and hydroquinone all together. Ultimately, I've found laser to be the most effective solution, but I may be biased because I see frustrated patients who have already tried topical treatments and are upset because they haven't worked for them. Topical medications are definitely worth a try and may work for you, but it's comforting to know that lasers are an option if they don't do the trick.

the problem: Eczema

WHAT IS IT, AND WHY DOES IT HAPPEN?

Eczema is a genetic type of rash that makes the skin sensitive and extremely dry and rough. A person can also have a temporary eczematic reaction to medication, an irritating substance, or an internal illness. Eczema frequently occurs in babies and toddlers, but luckily children usually grow out of the condition. This kind of eczema is called atopic dermatitis. It is the classic form of the disease and manifests as either rough bumps on the cheeks and arms (keratosis pilaris), dry and red patches in the creases of the elbows and knees, or fissures behind the earlobes and on eyelid creases.

HOW CAN I PREVENT IT?

Dry skin is the issue, so moisturize at least twice a day with a rich, occlusive cream or ointment. Slather on greasy moisturizer (a regular body lotion is not enough) as soon as you dry off after the shower. Wait five minutes for the cream to sink in and put on another coat. You can't moisturize eczema too much. Avoid long, hot baths or showers that dehydrate the skin. Don't try to scrub off the dry eczematic skin, and don't use water or alcohol-based products that dry it out. Strong detergents, harsh acids, and active ingredients and perfumes can all aggravate the condition. Sweat irritates it too, so be sure to cleanse the skin soon after a workout. If you're sleeping in an overheated room, crack open a window so you don't get too warm, and wear cotton clothing to absorb perspiration. Use a humidifier to add moisture to the air if your bedroom is especially dry. It can be a completely dehydrating environment in winter when the radiator is blasting.

HOW CAN I TREAT IT MYSELF?

Besides vigilant moisturizing, you can try an OTC cortisone cream. But to be honest, a 1% concentration probably isn't going to do much for you. It's best to get a prescription steroid from your doctor.

E

WHAT CAN A DOCTOR DO?

I usually prescribe a topical, not an oral, medication. A prescription topical steroid or a topical nonsteroidal anti-inflammatory—such as tacrolimus (Protopic) or pimecrolimus (Elidel)—reduce inflammation, relieve itching, and moisturize the skin. Steroids may be safer options for treating babies and children because they're time-tested. A patient with moderate to severe eczema must calm the rashy inflammation down and shouldn't worry too much about using a topical steroid. Patients use it temporarily, twice daily for one to two weeks. With mild eczema—normal skin that may have an itchy, dry patch or two—a nonsteroidal anti-inflammatory should work fine and won't have steroid side effects such as thinning or atrophied skin. (These effects happen only with long-term use of topical steroids.)

>>> q&a

Q: What are the rough bumps on my upper arms? My son seems to have the same thing on his cheeks. Is it rosacea or a rash?

A: It's neither. Both of you have keratosis pilaris, which is a form of eczema. Instead of round bumps, dry skin can make triangular, pyramid-shaped bumps, or accuminate papules. The keratin on top is shaped like a sharp spike, which is why the skin is so rough. There's no good reason why these bumps are triangular while others elsewhere are round. Keratosis pilaris is usually found on the upper arms, the upper lateral thighs, and (especially on children) the cheeks. Like most eczema, the genetic condition stems from dry, sensitive skin and tends to get worse in the winter, when it's cold and dry. Ironically, most people with KP tend to do just the opposite of what they should to treat the condition. They avoid moisturizing the area (thinking it's a form of acne), when what's really needed is the thickest cream possible.

The best prevention is slathering on a rich cream or ointment (one that contains occlusive emollients such as petrolatum, lanolin, and mineral oil) regularly to moisturize and protect the skin. You can't apply too much. It will help keep the condition in check and may help it go away. (My stepson has KP on his cheeks, and I chase him around constantly trying to put more moisturizer on his face.) When skin is chronically dehydrated, it tries to heal itself and the natural pattern of exfoliation is disrupted. For this reason, you can use a loofah or body brush to gently scrub off the dead skin cells. I also recommend over-the-counter lotions such as Lac-Hydrin or AmLactin to be applied once or twice a day. They contain lactic acid (a great gentle exfoliant for sensitive skin) in a moisturizing base. Another effective treatment is a retinoid lotion, which regulates keratinocyte turnover and helps slough off the heaped-up, pointy dead skin cells. To accelerate the exfoliation process, a dermatologist can do microdermabrasion and a light chemical peel followed by a deep moisturizing mask. Once the area is smooth, a field of tiny red dots will be left behind. They will fade somewhat though probably not completely) on their own. A pulsed dye laser treatment can make the redness go away faster.

If the area becomes raw and red, a doctor can prescribe an antibiotic lotion or a topical steroid cream. Often I simply recommend an over-the-counter topical antibiotic, a first-aid ointment such as Neosporin.

>>> skin lie: Enlarged pores are abnormal.

>>> skin truth: Most of the time what we consider enlarged pores are hair follicles on the nose or chin. It's common to confuse perfectly normal pores with open comedones, or blackheads, but they are not synonymous. A blackhead is a pore that's plugged with keratin. A normal pore is basically a pinhole opening in the skin, either a sweat gland or a follicle, that probably contains a tiny hair or some healthy white keratin inside. These are frequently mistaken for something bad, such as bacteria or dirt. Not so.

I bet you have one of those magnifying mirrors in your bathroom that makes everything on your face, including regular pores, ten times bigger. I tell many patients to throw away that mirror. It leads to so many extra, unnecessary purchases, such as products that claim to "deep clean," "purify," and "tighten" pores. It is not physically possible to do any of these things. These products essentially strip out the keratin that lives in the pore, so it's momentarily empty and may appear to be smaller for a little while—but it will eventually fill up again. Again, it's perfectly normal to have keratin, sebum, or a minuscule hair inside a pore. It's part of the skin's defense barrier to have that oil and keratin in the pores since it prevents bacteria from occupying that space.

If your pores appear to be dilated, first see your dermatologist to be sure that you don't have rosacea or acne, conditions that could be mistaken for enlarged pores and should be treated with medication. Then think about why your pores look enlarged. Is it genetic? In which case, pretty much nothing is going to change them. Do you have dry skin, which when moisturized can plump up and make the pores look smaller? Are you prone to comedones (cystlike blackheads or whiteheads), which are not technically enlarged pores but can be improved with regular exfoliation or retinoids? More often than not, a dilated pore is due to sun damage. What does one have to do with the other? Consider that pores require the structural base of collagen and elastin to hold them nice and tight. When that foundation is vaporized over time by ultraviolet radiation (or aging), the pores can appear more open, a condition known as "patulous pores." If sun damage or the aging process is the reason behind large pores, my job is to try to build the collagen back up again with methods like laser, microdermabrasion, or chemical peels. (I will discuss photo rejuvenation techniques such as this in chapter 10.)

>>> q&a

Q: Are freckles dangerous?

A: I don't consider freckles to be a problem and they aren't dangerous, but they are a marker of sun damage. How many freckles someone has tells me how much sun exposure he or she has had. Freckles are usually an indication that someone is at higher risk of skin cancer (since they are usually found on people with lighter skin and eyes), but darker skin can freckle too. You aren't usually born with freckles; they develop in the sun.

Patients often come in who want their freckles erased. If there are a few that stand out, or to decrease the overall number, I use a YAG or ruby laser (the kinds that target pigment) to get rid of them. These lasers are specific (about the size of a pen) and zap essentially one freckle at a time. They also leave a scab, so I wouldn't want to vaporize an entire face. Although I don't recommend it, I have had three patients insist that I treat their freckles head to toe—probably more than a thousand spots! It's time-consuming, expensive, and overwhelming for the patient, and the recovery time for something as extensive as that would be at least one month.

the problem: Hair Loss

WHAT A DOCTOR CALLS IT: alopecia (hair loss that can be scarring or nonscarring) or telogen effluvium (nonscarring, temporary hair loss)

WHAT IS IT, AND WHY DOES IT HAPPEN?
Telogen effluvium, which is temporary, diffuse hair loss, commonly occurs due to stress or physical trauma, and it's often associated with hormonal imbalances. It can happen after having a baby or as a result of an illness, surgery, or emotional turmoil. Hair growth and shedding happen in three phases—the anagen, or growth phase; the catagen, or transition stage; and the telogen or resting phase. A shock to the system can cause these growth cycles to reset at the same time so a much larger number of hairs falls out simultaneously. During pregnancy, your hair gets fuller (like everything else in your body, it's growing at a rapid rate), so it may seem that you're losing more strands than normal six months after giving birth, but the hair is probably simply going back to its normal prepregnancy thickness. (This happened to

me, and it's disconcerting to see all that hair in the shower drain. The truth is, my hair did go back to its normal texture, but it took over two years!)

Androgenetic alopecia is progressive hair loss due to hormonal changes such as menopause. It is nonscarring but still very distressing. Hair dissipates in the center, in a Christmas tree pattern, and this happens as hormones wane and the strand caliber reverts to that of weaker, vellus hair. The gradual thinning is similar to that in male-pattern baldness (although in men the condition may be more genetic than hormonal. Thyroid problems, certain medications, anemia, psoriasis, and vitamin deficiencies can all contribute to hair loss, or alopecia. It's important to see a dermatologist who can do a workup and test you for any serious health problems that can narrow down the cause. The doctor will do a simple blood test or a punch biopsy of the scalp to establish a diagnosis.

There are also other forms of hair loss, including alopecia areata, an autoimmune disorder in which the immune system attacks the hair follicles, and traction alopecia, when hair falls out from being pulled back too tightly on a regular basis. Harsh hair-straightening treatments (ones using chemicals such as formaldehyde) can make hair fall out too.

WHAT CAN I DO TO PREVENT IT, AND HOW CAN I TREAT IT MYSELF?
In the case of telogen effluvium, it's more of a waiting process for the growth cycle to go back to normal. Some believe that biotin or vitamin B12 shots can help, but I'm of the opinion that a healthy diet sans supplements is sufficient. Minoxidil (Rogaine) has been very effective at halting more hair loss, but there's one caveat: when you stop using the product, your hair starts shedding again. In the case of temporary loss, minoxidil can maintain the hair you have until the body gets back to normal, and then you can stop using it.

New at-home laser light gadgets claim to stimulate hair follicles to go into a growth phase and reduce inflammation that might be inhibiting hair growth. But there is absolutely no strong science to back up these claims.

WHAT CAN A DOCTOR DO?

Not all dermatologists specialize in hair loss, but most are capable of getting you started by determining a diagnosis. The doctor may do a biopsy, have blood work done, and can refer you to a specialist. A prescription for topical minoxidil (Rogaine) can help, and finasteride (Propecia, an oral medication originally developed for blood pressure) has been proven effective for male-pattern baldness but is not safe for women since it can cause birth defects. Both medications help stimulate new growth in the hair follicle and diminish the progression of hair loss. In cases of alopecia and male-pattern baldness that become worse, it's comforting to know that hair transplants are a terrific solution. They now grow in naturally and are better than ever before.

the problem: An Ingrown Hair

WHAT IS IT?

When a hair gets trapped and starts growing underneath the skin, it can create a bump and cause folliculitis, an inflammation of the hair follicle. Inflammatory cells (neutrophils) race to the area to kill bacteria around the jagged ingrown hair that is penetrating the follicular wall. This neutrophilic accumulation causes a small papule, or pimple.

WHY DOES IT HAPPEN?

An ingrown hair occurs when a hair is either broken off (tweezed or waxed) or cut off at the very surface of the skin with a razor. The hair can grow back at an angle and miss the opening of the follicle, curl back around, and become captured under the skin. Ingrown hairs are more common in those with curly, coarse hair. Some dark-skinned men suffer from a condition called acne keloidalis, in which ingrown hairs on the face or neck turn into keloids, or raised scars.

HOW CAN I PREVENT IT?

Men and women who are prone to ingrown hairs may want to avoid the close shave that causes the problem. Some men find that an electric razor doesn't cut as close, and shaving with the grain of the hair helps too. There's also a special razor blade called the Bump Fighter designed specifically to prevent this problem by keeping the blade slightly above the skin level so it can't cut hair off too closely.

Regular exfoliation can help prevent ingrown hairs by keeping the follicles open so they can't trap hairs in the first place. Salicylic acid (in a toner or a pad), a loofah, or a washcloth works well. Because these hairs can get stuck deep under the skin, salicylic or glycolic acid isn't enough once the ingrown hair is trapped. Don't exfoliate if you already have an inflamed ingrown hair—it will only cause trauma to the area.

HOW CAN I TREAT IT MYSELF?

It's very difficult to get rid of an ingrown hair yourself. Scrubbing or trying to extricate the hair yourself usually leads to infection and frustration. If an ingrown hair becomes embedded and inflamed, use an over-the-counter disinfecting surgical scrub such as Hibiclens antiseptic cleanser, which contains chlorhexidine, to prevent infection. Applying the cleanser with a damp washcloth gently exfoliates the skin and may help release the hair.

WHAT CAN A DOCTOR DO?

Chronic ingrown hairs, especially if they become infected and inflamed, are grounds for laser hair removal. It's a wonderful option, even for men. It may take ten sessions to do a man's face and three to eight for a woman's bikini line, but the process will put a stop to ingrown hairs forever. Men can then cut shaving down to once every four days, which greatly decreases the occurrence of both razor burn and bumps.

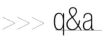

Q: How can I help my husband not to get razor burn from shaving?

A: Razor burn is an abrasion caused by the blade scraping against the skin. Your husband is not alone. A 2005 poll conducted by the American Academy of Dermatology found that 78 percent of men who shave have experienced irritation. It's very common and usually happens on sensitive skin (such as a man's face or neck or a woman's underarms). The culprit is almost always a dull razor blade, since you need to use more pressure to get the shaving done. (Replace the blade every two to four shaves; some men might need to replace it every time.) Along with using a fresh, sharp blade, your husband should apply enough shaving cream to keep his skin protected and lubricated as the razor slides across it. A lot of men make their razor burn worse when they put on after-shave right after abrading it. These astringent products usually contain alcohol or menthol, which makes irritated skin sting and become even more inflamed. Better to use a soothing, anti-inflammatory moisturizer containing aloe, allantoin, or chamomile. When an area is especially painful, a topical steroid cream can be applied to calm inflammation.

the problem: Melasma

WHAT IS IT?
Melasma is a tan, symmetrical, and very stubborn patch of hyperpigmentation, usually found on the cheekbones, forehead, and upper lip. It can be a big blotchy mark or a small dark stain. If you have a similar discoloration on both sides of the mouth or both cheeks, that fits the pattern of melasma.

WHY DOES IT HAPPEN?
Estrogen seems to be the primary instigator here, which is why melasma is often called "the mask of pregnancy." (Only 10 percent of

M

those affected are men, according to the American Academy of Dermatology.) It happens frequently to expectant mothers and shows up when a woman goes on birth control pills. Hormone-related melasma sometimes disappears by itself six months after giving birth or if you stop taking birth control pills with a high estrogen level. If hormones start the pigmentation ball rolling, UV exposure certainly runs with it. You cannot get melasma without the sun—it triggers super-sensitive melanocytes to accelerate production.

HOW CAN I PREVENT IT?

Have your hormone status checked by a doctor, and protect yourself from the sun. Sunscreen is the best prevention for any kind of hyperpigmentation, including melasma. You can try any remedy, and nothing will work if you keep going out in the sun. And if you begin using hydroquinone or retinoids, be even more vigilant with sun protection, since these medications make skin photosensitive. It's almost impossible to avoid melasma if you are prone to it, but do your best with sunscreen.

HOW CAN I TREAT IT MYSELF?

Think of melasma as a big brown spot, so treating it with the same kind of lightening agent—kojic, lactic, glycolic, or azeleic acid or hydroquinone—can be effective. I like to prescribe a cream with the trifecta of hydroquinone, topical steroid, and retinoid to be applied to the area once or twice a day until the pigmentation is gone (or less than a year). This plus the conscientious use of sunscreen can remedy the problem over a span of months.

WHAT CAN A DOCTOR DO?

There are various types of melasma, depending on how deep they are in the skin. When it is diagnosed, the dermatologist will use a Wood's lamp to enhance the pigment. If the hyperpigmentation looks even darker under the light, it's probably deeper in the skin and will be harder to treat.

Most melasma is superficial, and the best treatment (in addition to prescription lightening creams) is a 20% to 30% TCA or Jessner's chemical peel. I do a 30% peel on myself twice a year to keep my melasma at bay. A glycolic acid peel can be done on people with darker or more sensitive skin, since it's gentler than trichloroacetic acid (TCA). Both are melanotoxic and can decrease the number of melanocytes in the area for good. Usually one to three peels (followed by micro-dermabrasion seven to ten days after the peel) gets rid of the hyperpig-mentation, although the success rate varies from person to person.

For deeper melasma, my best prescription is two chemical peels a year and two to four Fraxel laser resurfacing treatments per year to get rid of both the superficial and the deeper pigment. Fraxel essentially removes pigment through intense exfoliation (in the same way it's used for stretch marks). (See "Stretch Marks" on page 242.) The laser heat basically drills microscopic pinholes through the skin and vaporizes whatever is in its path. This creates a controlled wound that in turn causes a fast reconstruction of the skin, so the healing process is fairly quick (usually about thirty-six hours). It's important to remember that melasma is a maintenance issue, and people go through years of the discoloration coming and going. This is a case where upkeep and pre-vention (in the form of sun protection) is key.

the problem: Moles

WHAT A DOCTOR CALLS THEM: benign melanocytic nevi

WHAT ARE THEY?
There are three general types of moles. One type is a flat, dark brown spot (a benign melanocytic nevus), another is pigmented and slightly raised (a junctional nevus), and there are also flesh-colored bumpy moles (intradermal nevi). Robert Redford has intradermal nevi, Sarah Jessica Parker had a junctional nevus on her chin (which recently was

M

surgically removed), Cindy Crawford has a junctional nevus near her lip, and Marilyn Monroe had a very famous benign melanocytic nevus. It's no wonder these are known as "beauty marks."

WHY DO THEY HAPPEN?

A nevus is a nest of cells that grows larger or more protuberant as we age. This group of skin cells is so tiny that it usually doesn't show up as a visible mole until about the age of four. When melanocytes are mixed into the nevus, it will appear pigmented.

HOW CAN I PREVENT THEM?

Benign melanocytic nevi show up on the skin naturally; and some—called congenital nevi—are evident at birth. They are part of your own personal skin topography and can't be avoided.

HOW CAN I TREAT THEM MYSELF?

Because melanocytic nevi are benign, they don't need to be addressed at all. One caveat: because we know that a skin cancer sometimes mimics a benign-appearing lesion, you should be conscientious about regular skin checks and watch for changes in the appearance of existing moles.

WHAT CAN A DOCTOR DO?

Most benign moles don't need to be taken off unless they bother you aesthetically. There are two relatively easy methods of removal. A raised nevus can be sculpted flat using electrodessication, essentially burning off the top surface so it's even with the skin. The problem with this approach is that a portion of the mole is still left under the skin, so it has a fifty-fifty chance of repigmenting within a year. (It usually remains flat, however). The surefire way to get rid of a mole forever is to excise it, although you may be trading that little mole for a tiny scar (left from the stitch that's required)—although most often the scar will completely vanish in a couple months.

the problem: Psoriasis

WHAT IS IT?

This condition is characterized by thick, red plaque with a white, silvery (micaceous) scale on top. It's itchy and painful and can create big fissures on the skin. It tends to be on extensor surfaces, such as the elbows, knees, and scalp. There are several types of psoriasis, and some can be quite severe, affecting the joints and causing something called "psoriatic arthritis." It can also be mild, manifesting itself as one patch of plaque on the body, such as dry, cracked elbows that don't soften no matter how much moisturizer you put on.

WHY DOES IT HAPPEN?

Psoriasis is a genetic, chronic inflammatory disease where for some reason the lymphocytes (immune cells) are attacking the skin, causing cell turnover to accelerate. Therefore, the dead skin cells aren't shedding as fast as the maturing cells are rising to the surface. This pile-up creates a silvery scale on the surface.

WHAT CAN I DO TO PREVENT IT, AND HOW CAN I TREAT IT MYSELF?

Don't scratch or try to scrub off the scaly skin. Instead, moisturize with a thick, occlusive cream or ointment twice a day. Sweat will irritate the skin, as will fragranced products or perfume. Psoriasis sufferers have to be careful about everything they put on their skin—even sunscreen can sting. Even one patch of plaque should lead you to see a dermatologist, especially since it's likely that you will develop others in the future. It's important to get onto a good treatment program to prevent a more extensive outbreak.

WHAT CAN A DOCTOR DO?

Psoriasis is treated topically with a strong steroid cream to reduce inflammation and a vitamin D–derived ointment or cream (calcipotriol) that works to slow cell turnover. Believe it or not, another effective prescription is 6% salicylic acid (compounded with petrolatum into an ointment), which should be applied to the affected area every day. It gently exfoliates the scaly surface so that the topical steroid can penetrate into the diseased skin. A patient does see rapid improvement but must use these medications regularly to keep the condition under control.

Phototherapy, using UVB light to treat psoriasis inflammation, is still used, although it does have side effects of photodamage and an increased risk of skin cancer. Basically, the patient stands inside a walk-in light box for thirty seconds to nine minutes three times per week. The UV radiation, administered in metered doses, acts as an anti-inflammatory and immunosuppressant. A handheld UVB laser such as Excimer has also been used with great success for plaque psoriasis and doesn't expose the whole body to radiation.

This is the golden age of psoriasis treatment. The development of new medications for psoriasis is one of the most advanced and exciting in the entire field of dermatology. In the past five years, a revolutionary immunotherapy has been successful for treating more severe cases of psoriasis. This entails twice-a-week infusions of antibodies (proteins that lock onto a cell and suppress it) to block lymphocytes from attacking the skin. This can now be prescribed as an at-home injection too. It has put many patients into remission for a long time. An FDA panel just voted to recommend approval of a new psoriasis drug called ustekinumab, which targets the immune system to reduce inflammation. Another systemic medication that works well for psoriasis is acitretin (Soriatane), a vitamin A derivative similar to Accutane. It helps regulate the cell turnover cycle. Because the side effects of these medications can be intense, a doctor will choose one rather than using combination therapy for psoriasis.

the problem: Puffy Eyes

WHAT A DOCTOR CALLS IT: periorbital edema

WHAT IS IT?

An edema is too much fluid in the skin tissue, in this case under the eyes. This water or fluid retention can be due to anything from too little sleep to too much salty food.

WHY DOES IT HAPPEN?

You are either retaining water or not draining it normally. Remember that sleeping puts the parasympathetic nervous system in control and allows peripheral vessels near the skin to open up, thus moving nutrients to the skin and draining fluid from it. Not getting enough sleep stops that process of normal fluid balancing from happening. Water retention shows up more in the skin, and especially under the eyes, but you are actually retaining fluid everywhere. Besides a lack of sleep, puffy eyes can be triggered by a sinus infection, a cold, or an allergy.

HOW CAN I PREVENT IT?

Get enough sleep, and avoid salty foods, which cause water retention. Elevating your head with an extra pillow may help gravity along in the drainage process. Make sure that your puffiness isn't an inflammatory reaction to a skin care product, and see your ophthalmologist to rule out an anatomical symptom of something more serious. (Protuberant eyes, or exophthalmos, can be a sign of a thyroid disorder, for example.)

HOW CAN I TREAT IT MYSELF?

Something as simple as massaging the area helps move extra fluid away from it. This method manually distributes the fluid to other blood vessels, which can then drain it. There are plenty of home remedies for this particular problem, and, surprisingly, some of them actually might work. A cold compress isn't going to make a major change, but the cold does cause temporary vasoconstriction of the blood vessels. (Although once you remove the compress, the vessels dilate again.) Slices of cucumber may have an anti-inflammatory effect, but it's likely that the chill of the cucumber is more helpful. It's believed that products containing caffeine may constrict the blood vessels and reduce swelling. This seems highly unlikely, since caffeine is probably not able to penetrate to the vessels. Preparation H, the hemorrhoid cream, is supposed to work in a similar way (and there are lots of fashion models who supposedly use this trick). A little facial massage sounds like a more appealing, and definitely safer, choice to me and probably works just as well.

WHAT CAN A DOCTOR DO?
Puffy eyes are usually temporary and don't require a doctor visit. If the problem persists or seems to worsen, a dermatologist can determine if you have either fat herniations or malar festoons. A fat herniation is when the fat pad under the eye shifts out of place. A malar festoon is a semicircle of swelling that looks like a puffy banner under the eye and upper cheekbone. It's caused when circulatory problems obstruct the drainage of fluid. Both festoons and fat herniations can be corrected with cosmetic surgery. Bags or puffiness under the eyes can be diminished by injecting a dermal filler into the triangular hollow between the lower eyelid and the top of the cheek near the nose (the tear trough), which improves the eyelid-to-cheek contour so that the demarcation isn't so pronounced. (See chapter 10 for more information on fillers under the eyes.)

R

34 Ellen Marmur, MD

the problem: Rosacea

WHAT IS IT?

A hypersensitivity to sun and other factors cause blood vessels near the skin to dilate. This rush of circulation makes the complexion appear red and sets off a vicious cycle of inflammatory cells rushing to the area and triggering angiogenesis (the growth of more blood vessels). The body's wound-healing response tries to provide more highways, or veins, so inflammatory cells can go fix the problem near the skin, and consequently creates a bigger problem. Like acne, rosacea has a diagnostic spectrum of mild to severe. It can generate mild flushing, persistent redness, or the more severe papular kind of acne rosacea with bumpy pimples and sometimes thickening of the skin (rhinophyma). Those tiny pink papules contain inflammatory cells (neutrophils or T-cells), just like the pimples caused by dry skin or irritation.

WHY DOES IT HAPPEN, AND HOW CAN I PREVENT IT?

This genetic inflammatory disorder has no known cause and is especially common for those with fair skin and light eyes. The triggers, however, are well known, and avoiding them is key to alleviating the problem. Chief among them is UV exposure, and the cheapest, easiest, and most effective way to treat rosacea is to wear sunscreen and stay out of the sun. Heat (and hot, spicy food) is another trigger, so it's important to keep your temperature regulated. Try not to take long, hot showers or baths, and exercise in a cool environment (swimming is a good sport for people with rosacea). If you begin to heat up and start to flush, drink a glass of ice water to cool you down from the inside out.

HOW CAN I TREAT IT MYSELF?

Always wear sunblock, and know your personal rosacea triggers so you can avoid them. Gravitate toward using anti-redness cleanser and a moisturizer that contains anti-inflammatory ingredients such as al-

R

lantoin, aloe, or chamomile. Anyone with moderate to severe rosacea should see a dermatologist, who can get this chronic situation under control with medications.

WHAT CAN A DOCTOR DO?

A doctor can prescribe a topical antibiotic such as metronidazole (MetroGel), which works as a powerful anti-inflammatory, or Finacea, made from azelaic acid, which has anti-inflammatory properties, to control symptoms. Finacea is used for the papular, bumpy kind of rosacea, but it can be too strong for some people. Sulfa medications (lotion or cleansing pads) also work as anti-inflammatory antidotes. New low-dose oral antibiotics such as Oracea provide another way to reduce inflammation but don't have the antimicrobial properties or side effects of stronger antibiotics. I often combine low-dose systemic medication with the topicals (MetroGel or a sulfa-based lotion) for moderate or severe conditions. Another magic bullet is a low dose of a beta-blocker such as propranolol, a systemic medication designed for high blood pressure that helps prevent vasodilation and its ensuing redness. (I've used this for many blushing brides with great success.) Doctors don't prescribe topical steroids for rosacea. Though they can calm it initially, steroids cause a rebound rosacea flare-up soon after you stop applying the medication.

Intense pulsed light (IPL) treatments augment topical or systemic medications by eliminating the superficial blood vessels that contribute to flushing. As with acne, if someone is seeing me for rosacea I start with medications first and then move on to procedures that target inflammation. I've found IPL to be absolutely the most effective light or laser therapy for rosacea because it eradicates extra vessels (by inducing apoptosis, or programmed cell death) without causing bruising and with relatively no downtime or discomfort. IPL can disintegrate thousands of blood vessels at once with its larger, broad surface, whereas a vascular beam laser, which is shaped like a pen, gets fewer at a time. I use Vbeam for cases of severe rosacea, when I need a more powerful machine to tackle stronger and bigger vessels. Most patients need about five treatments spaced out by three to six weeks. It takes at least three sessions for the IPL to kill off enough blood vessels to see a difference. (I've had about five treatments myself to quell my own rosacea problem.) Eventually rosacea is bound to return, but if you're diligent with sun protection and avoid your triggers, positive results will last a lot longer.

the problem: A Scar

WHAT IS IT?

There are five types of scars. Some scars present as post-inflammatory hypo- or hyperpigmentation (PIH). Hyperpigmentation is a brown stain on the skin, and hypopigmentation is a white mark that tends to be permanent. This occurs because inflammation from a trauma can stimulate the melanocytes to make too much melanin. Pitted scars are indented and often occur after chicken pox or acne. Normal scars are firm. This type of scar is a bundle of extra, abnormally constructed collagen that arises as a result of trauma to the skin. Normally collagen is woven together horizontally, but because a scar grows too fast and with no organization, it creates a huge, haphazard knot. The fourth type is a hypertrophic scar that is raised and firm, but the same size as the original wound. Finally, the fifth type of scar is a keloid, which grows beyond the original size of the wound. It often occurs on the earlobe or the chest.

HOW CAN I PREVENT IT?

Basic wound healing is the best prevention. Proper healing requires a slightly moist environment in which the cells can replicate and connect to each other properly. Clean the wound twice a day with soap and water, apply an antibiotic ointment (such as Polysporin or Neosporin), and cover it with a bandage. And never pick or scratch at a scab. This sounds obvious, but people do it all the time. By pulling off the skin, you are actually ripping off the dermis, and that leads to a scar. By the way, the old wives' tale of putting vitamin E on a scar or a scab is just that. How a wound heals is what generates a scar, and moisturizing the skin after the fact won't do too much in the way of prevention. It's not the vitamin E but the oily texture that helps.

WHAT CAN A DOCTOR DO?

The art of scar revision is complex, and most of the time the best we can do is improve its appearance. I always tell my patients, "It will look better, but it won't be perfect." Rarely can we make a scar disappear completely. There are as many remedies as there are scars, and each variation requires a specific treatment. Raised keloid and hypertrophic scars can be treated with a series of hydrocortisone injections that help shrink the collagen. Keloids are often very red, so a Vbeam laser can knock out the vessels that are feeding the scar, diminishing redness and shrinking the bulk even more. This process requires three to five sessions. Dermabrasion, a technique to vaporize the skin by way of electrocautery or ablative lasers (such as CO_2 or erbium: YAG lasers), can remove raised scars. (My main use of dermabrasion is for scar revision, rather than for any antiaging procedure.) First I use a numbing cream and inject a touch of lidocaine into the area. Then I use an electric pen to literally burn off the scar with heat.

Postinflammatory hyperpigmentation is usually deep in the dermis, and for some reason lasers for pigment (ruby and Nd:YAG) aren't very successful because they work best on superficial pigment. Fractionated laser resurfacing works better on darker brown, white, or red scars. It essentially vaporizes the pigment and exfoliates the scar from the skin. The patient requires about four treatments and will see a 50 to 80 percent improvement.

the problem: Seborrheic Keratosis

WHAT IS IT?

This benign lesion is a dry, raised, wart-like growth that appears on the skin seemingly overnight and out of nowhere. It is easily mistaken for a scab that forms over a pimple that's healing, but this one won't go away. The growth is created when too many dead keratinocytes get rolled up like an onion into a scaly little mass, which is why it looks and feels like a hard clay blob. Seborrheic keratoses (SK) have been dubbed "keratin pearls," but they're stuck onto the skin more like a barnacle.

WHY DOES IT HAPPEN?

It's simple genetic programming and another irritating aspect of aging. Some people make different spots as they get older. I make milia (which I discussed earlier in this chapter), but many people make seborrheic keratoses. They are painless but have dogged staying power—since they are stuck like glue to the skin, they can be extremely annoying.

HOW CAN I PREVENT OR TREAT IT AT HOME?

Unfortunately, there is nothing you can do to prevent an SK and nothing you can do yourself to get rid of it. It seems as if you could scratch it right off, but trust me, as annoying as it is, you can scrub all you want and that little keratin blob won't budge.

WHAT CAN A DOCTOR DO?

Dermatologists use one of several methods to remove a seborrheic keratosis. Liquid nitrogen can take it off (although that can ultimately leave a tiny white spot), or it can be scraped off with a curette. I prefer to use electrocautery to sculpt the growth off. Local anesthetic is injected into the area first, and then it takes just a few seconds to remove it with an electric pen. The procedure leaves an abrasion, a little pink spot that will eventually go away, and the area will regrow normal skin. Hopefully that growth will never come back, but you are destined to get others.

S

the problem: Skin Tags

WHAT A DOCTOR CALLS IT: acrochordon

WHAT ARE THEY?

A skin tag is a small, fleshy, raised growth of all the layers of the skin, including the dermis. Almost all the time, skin tags are totally benign. Skin tags sometimes appear darker than your normal skin tone because the skin is squished together and pigment is concentrated into this tiny area. They usually occur on the neck and upper and lower eyelids, in the groin area, and in the underarms.

WHY DO THEY HAPPEN?

Like so many other skin conditions, skin tags are genetic. They happen in places of wear and tear and show up where skin (or items such as clothing or jewelry) rub against skin, for instance on the neck or underarms. For this reason, obesity can make them worse. Skin tags tend to increase during pregnancy, when everything in the body grows at an accelerated rate. Sometimes pregnancy skin tags go away by themselves about six months after a woman gives birth. Most of the time, however, skin tags have to be removed by a doctor.

HOW CAN I PREVENT THEM?

There is no way to prevent or treat skin tags at home. Losing weight may help if the cause is obesity.

HOW CAN I TREAT THEM MYSELF?

Unfortunately, there is no way to get rid of skin tags yourself—and please don't attempt to! Patients have come to me after tying strings around their skin tags to suffocate the growth. This doesn't work and can cause a staphylococcus infection.

WHAT CAN A DOCTOR DO?

A dermatologist removes a skin tag in one of three ways: by surgically snipping it off, burning it off with electrocauterization (if the tag is tiny), or freezing it off with liquid nitrogen. I usually choose the first method. First I inject a local anesthetic at the base of the skin tag; then I use forceps and scissors to remove it. Because there's usually a blood vessel inside the skin tag, it can bleed more than you would think when it's removed. And because nerves are contained in the skin tag, excision is painful and the injection of lidocaine is essential. All three of these methods leave a scab that heals within a week or two. I have patients who come in once every year or two to get their skin tags cleaned up. After excision, doctors routinely send larger skin tags to the pathology lab to check for melanoma, although the chance of malignancy is extremely rare.

the problem: Spider Veins on the Face

WHAT A DOCTOR CALLS THEM: telangiectasia

WHAT ARE THEY?

These are normal, superficial, and far too obvious veins—arterial offshoots of the bigger, robust artery that goes up the nose and the middle of the face. That's why they are usually right near the nostrils. These arterials aren't necessarily broken or dilated; they're just close to the surface.

WHY DO THEY HAPPEN?

What can I say? They just show up, and near the surface of the skin is somewhere for them to go. As we age, we grow more and more of these fine vessels through a vascular growth process called angiogenesis. At the same time we lose fat and the skin becomes more translucent as the years go on, so these arterials become more evident. People with hay fever and allergies tend to have more irritation around the nose, and this might cause extra blood vessels to grow there. Genetics is a factor, and sun damage makes them worse by dissolving the collagen around the vessels that usually camouflage them and by causing inflammation, which revs up angiogenesis.

HOW CAN I PREVENT IT?
Unfortunately, there's no great way to prevent these veins from showing up. Sun protection can help, and treatments for rosacea (topical anti-inflammatory gels and creams) may calm the redness because angiogenesis occurs as a result of an inflammatory response (the body builds more highways to help inflammatory cells travel to an irritated or inflamed area).

HOW CAN I TREAT IT MYSELF?
Lots of magazine articles tout the claim that topical vitamin K can somehow diminish spider veins. I don't think this vitamin (taken orally by people with liver problems and those whose blood does not clot properly) can do much when applied to the skin to affect the appearance of surface blood vessels. Knowing your skin and its triggers is the key because, similar to rosacea, avoiding flushing is half the battle.

WHAT CAN A DOCTOR DO?
Removal is tricky because these tiny branches are attached to a larger, forceful artery. Because of the high blood flow, they can be very resistant. For me, the gold standard of treatment for spider veins on the face is the Vbeam pulsed dye laser. It heats up the blood inside the vessel, and when that heat dissipates it fries the vessel wall. Then scavenger cells called macrophages come in and gobble up the dead vein like garbage. (Since there are plenty of working veins a little bit deeper in the skin, it's completely safe to destroy the superficial ones.) The procedure takes about twenty minutes, and three to five laser treatments are usually necessary to weaken the vessels enough without exploding them and causing a bruise. Because these veins are connected

to a large artery, it's hard to get them to disappear forever. Think of laser treatments as upkeep that you may need to repeat every couple years.

the problem: Stretch Marks

WHAT A DOCTOR CALLS THEM: striae gravidarum (pregnancy stretch marks), striae albae (white stretch marks), or striae rubrae (red stretch marks)

WHAT ARE THEY?

Stretch marks are technically atrophic scars, meaning the skin is thinner and pulled. They look like wiggly rivers with a slight indentation, almost like wood grain. The skin also tends to be a little shinier in the area. People usually get them around the belly, on the backs of the hips, on the insides of the knees, and on the sides of the breasts. Stretch marks tend to be symmetrical and localized, occurring on both hips, both knees, or both breasts.

WHY DO THEY HAPPEN?

These scars form when skin has lost the integrity and strong structure beneath it. Abnormal architecture of the collagen and elastin fibers in the dermis is the crux of the problem. During pregnancy the problem is twofold, since the skin is also stretched to the limit and doesn't return to its original, tight elasticity. Ultimately, stretch marks are genetic, so it's not true that only overweight or pregnant women get them. I've seen young women and those with model-thin physiques with them. Men get stretch marks (and steroid supplements increase the risk), and a lot of adolescents get them when hormones kick in and they have growth spurts. Though there's no typical stretch mark patient, rapid weight loss and gain are big factors.

HOW CAN I PREVENT THEM?

Because genetics is a strong factor, stretch marks are difficult to prevent. Moisturizing the skin and avoiding large weight loss or gain may help. Some women swear by using lubricating oils and ointments on the belly during their pregnancy. My obstetrician used a special type of oil during her own and did not develop stretch marks. Perhaps it worked by moisturizing the skin, or she might just be genetically blessed.

HOW CAN I TREAT THEM MYSELF?

First, the bad news: there is no such thing as erasing stretch marks completely. All you can do is improve the appearance and make them less visible. Once these scars emerge, products such as stretch mark oils and "restructuring" creams and gels can't do much. (Although some pregnancy stretch marks go away on their own over time, this is not the case for many women.) Retinoids may help, mainly because they exfoliate the epidermis. I've prescribed them for my patients, but any change is slow to occur; it could take years to see a difference. That's because stretch marks aren't necessarily a problem of the cell renewal process and that's where retinoids work best. And since these scars are on the body, not the face, absorption of retinoids to the dermis, where collagen and elastin are located, might be harder to achieve.

WHAT CAN A DOCTOR DO?

Again, the problem is frustrating for both doctor and patient since the best we can do is to diminish the appearance. Laser treatments are the best solution by far, but they involve a significant investment of time and money. Treating stretch marks requires a minimum of ten to twenty visits, and each can cost anywhere between $100 and $400. It adds up, and at best a patient may see a 50 to 80 percent improvement—which may be enough for people whose scars are very noticeable.

Striae rubrae are especially amenable to a pulsed dye laser (the Vbeam, which targets prominent blood vessels). When the texture of the scar is also an issue, I use a fractionated laser (such as Fraxel) for resurfacing the skin. It is essentially an extreme form of exfoliation, so the laser smoothes out the grooves on the skin in four to eight treatments. Fraxel has also been shown to improve the pigmentation of both white and red stretch marks, but I think it may be something of an illusion: the skin tone simply appears more even once the raised texture is improved. Striae albae the white, shiny scars, can be repigmented with an excimer laser, which emits UVB light that stimulates melanocytes to make more melanin in that area. It's almost like coloring with a crayon. I worked on a study with Dr. David Goldberg that proved that this UVB laser increased not only the number of melanocytes but also the size of the melanosomes they produced.[1]

There is a myth that stretch marks are harder to remove as they mature. This is not true. It is true that they usually start off as striae rubrae and mature into striae albae, but one is not worse or more difficult to treat than another. Unfortunately, they are equally hard to get rid of.

>>> q&a

Q: I'm considering getting my tattoo removed. How is this done, and is it painful?

A: Your change of heart is not uncommon. Twenty-four percent of Americans have at least one tattoo, and at least 17 percent seek to have them removed. A tattoo is similar to a scar that is deeply embedded in the dermis. The only way to remove one is through a series of laser treatments, and yes, it is painful. The important aspects of a tattoo, when it comes to removal, are the colors of ink involved and when it was placed on your skin. Surprisingly, older tattoos are easier to take off. A lot of military tattoos from more than thirty years ago were done with blue or black mineral inks, which tend to be more amenable to laser. The sophistication of the inks used now makes them more resistant to breaking down. They're much more permanent, and the colors used are more difficult to erase. Old-school blue and black inks are the easiest to remove because pigment-specific lasers, such as the ruby and YAG, target those dark colors successfully. Other colors have to be treated with a combination of lasers. Green ink responds only to the ruby laser, for example, and red responds only to the Nd:YAG. Sometimes the laser will actually convert the color of the tattoo through a chemical reaction, and ink that was red may turn black. Like scar revision, tattoo removal is not a perfect science. Depending on the colors and age of the tattoo, I can gauge how many sessions may be necessary to remove it. Usually it takes at least five treatments, and sometimes I've had to do up to seventeen. The procedure itself takes about ten minutes each time, and you have to return every six weeks for another one.

Laser removal of a tattoo is more painful than other laser treatments (such as those for getting rid of hair or brown spots) because the laser beam is shattering mineral ink particles deep in the dermis, after which the lymphatic system scavenges up the debris. We inject lidocaine first, but it's still not a pleasant ten-minute appointment. Afterward, the area blisters and scabs over. It's a wound, after all. Again, the final result depends on the colors and how lucky we are. I always warn patients that they'll probably have a trace shadow of the tattoo, and there's a possibility that you will be trading that tattoo for a scar.

An innovative new tattoo ink has just been developed that is much easier to laser off, perhaps in only one treatment. The Freedom-2 Infinitink is a biodegradable pigment encapsulated in plastic, a delivery system that allows the laser to hit its microscopic polymer beads, shatter them, and allow the dye to dissolve safely into the body. (The technology was originally developed by doctors in an effort to help cancer patients erase the tattooed markers used for radiation treatment.) So far, black ink is the only color on the market, but I'm sure that will change soon. It's a remarkable idea for those with a penchant for body art but a tendency to commitment-phobia.

the problem: Unwanted Hair

WHAT A DOCTOR CALLS IT: hypertrichosis

WHAT IS IT, AND WHY DOES IT HAPPEN?
Having too much hair in male patterns (on the abdomen or the face, for instance) is either hormonal or a normal ethnic variation. A lot of Greek, Italian, and Eastern European women have hypertrichosis to some extent. Many Asian women have dark peach fuzz (or vellus hairs) on their cheeks. Hair growth on the body starts in puberty and surges during pregnancy, and black hairs get thicker over time with age.

HOW CAN I TREAT IT MYSELF?
It seems that we are constantly trying to get rid of hair somewhere—legs, eyebrows, upper lip, underarms. There are plenty of at-home hair removal (or camouflaging) methods available at a spa or salon. We wage our battle with excess body hair with wax, razors, tweezers, threading, chemical depilatories, and facial bleach. All work to a certain degree, but all have their negatives. Waxing can cause postinflammatory hyperpigmentation, inflammatory papules, and folliculitis on some people. For most, it is totally safe. In fact, one could argue that waxing might even stimulate collagen production due to the slight trauma to the skin. The chemicals in depilatories can be extremely irritating to the skin and disintegrate hair only at the very surface. Bleaching hair on the skin is relatively safe but only camouflages the problem. Tweezing can leave ingrown hairs. The most glaring problem of all, however, is that none of these treatments eliminate hairs for good.

There are new at-home diode devices safe enough to use for do-it-yourself laser hair removal. Because they utilize relatively weak light sources, it takes a lot longer to see results compared to what you get at a doctor's office. Though these expensive gizmos can't replace the effectiveness of powerful lasers, they are a decent way to augment the laser hair removal a dermatologist does.

A relatively new weapon against hair regrowth is eflornithine hydrochloride (Vaniqa), a prescription topical hair inhibitor. It shrinks the hair bulb in the follicle and slows down the hair growth cycle. Some doctors use it to supplement laser hair removal treatments, and it definitely works. Once you stop using it, however, the speed of hair growth goes back to normal.

WHAT CAN A DOCTOR DO?

First a doctor will rule out any medical condition that may be causing hormonal hair growth. The growth of lots of vellus hair, for example, can be a sign of polycystic ovarian syndrome.

Dermatologists employ nonablative lasers (the kind that don't damage the epidermis) to dramatically reduce hair permanently. Most people see a reduction of 80 percent. (Some become 100 percent hair-free, but that's not the norm.) But hair is tenacious and continues to develop over time. Laser hair reduction is remarkably effective, depending upon the color of the patient's skin and hair and the texture of the hair. Because the laser zones in best on dark pigment in the hair matrix, the ideal patient has fair skin with dark hair. Lighter skin has less melanin to absorb the laser energy, and all the heat can go straight to the follicle without burning the skin. Coarse hair is also much easier for the laser to target since it's larger and has more pigment. Fair, fine hair doesn't respond well to laser removal. Because the laser energy targets melanin (in both the follicle and the skin), it can cause pigmentation problems for darker, more melanocytic complexions. For olive or darker skin tones, a laser with a longer wavelength and a longer pulse duration (such as an Nd:Yag) has less potential to harm or discolor the skin.

For people with fine hair that's either blond or red and won't respond to a laser, electrolysis is a viable option. A very fine needle is inserted into the individual hair follicle and emits an electric current that literally destroys it. The results are permanent, but the process is painstaking and painful. If you have three or four hairs or a small patch of hair to address, this can be a great alternative.

The genius of these lasers is that they can actually destroy something under the surface (such as hair in the follicle) without breaking the stratum corneum. For hair removal, I usually work with an alexandrite laser (which uses crystal to generate its laser light) or a diode (a super-conductor). IPL can also be successful but can take more treatments and may have more side effects for some people. It can also cause postinflammatory hyperpigmentation or hypopigmentation for those who are sensitive to IPL.

In many states it is illegal for spas and salons to use lasers, but they may use a light source such as IPL, often operated by a nonmedical aesthetician. Though some spas have a medical director on the premises, he or she may not even be a dermatologist. Not everyone gets successful results from IPL, and since different hair textures, colors, and skin tones require different kinds of lasers, it's important to have laser hair reduction administered by a fellowship-trained, laser-trained dermatologist.

WHAT HAPPENS BEFORE, DURING, AND AFTER LASER HAIR REDUCTION?
When you come in for a consultation, you should have some hair growth so the dermatologist can see the distribution of the hair and evaluate its caliber and color in order to assess what kind of laser to use. So don't shave for a week, and don't wax or bleach your upper lip beforehand. On the day of your laser treatment, you must be clean-shaven but not waxed. Hair stubble in the root will help capture the heat of the laser energy, but you don't want it above the skin because it will absorb laser energy you want reserved for the follicle. Numbing cream is applied for fifteen to twenty minutes and then carefully washed off. That takes the sting out of the laser, which feels like a hot rubber band snapping on the skin. As soon as an area is treated, little

black dots usually appear; this is stubble frying and rising to the surface. Sometimes it looks as if you have more hair after the session than before, but it will shed in the shower. These dots are replaced by red goose bumps (follicular edema). This is an effect we want to see, the clinical endpoint that shows the treatment worked. The red bumps are the result of the laser inducing folliculitis as a result of trauma to the follicle. This redness lasts from a few days to a week (and if those little black specks of stubble didn't shed before, they now come out).

Hair grows and sheds in stages, and a laser captures only hairs in the active growth phase, when the matrix is activated. Since only one third of hairs are affected at one time, most people require three to five treatments spaced at monthly intervals to take care of the other two thirds.

WHAT ARE THE SIDE EFFECTS?
Any kind of laser creates a controlled wound that revs up the inflammatory system to launch a response—in this case, scavenging the hair follicle. This can leave postinflammatory hyperpigmentation or hypopigmentation (white spots that arise on sensitive or darker skin). Any brown spots should be temporary and will fade away, but white spots may be permanent. They can be repigmented with an excimer laser. Occasionally a patient will get paradoxical hypertrichosis, which is more hair growth after laser treatment.[2] I've seen people who've had up to thirty sessions and felt that they were actually growing more hair. This may happen when the laser parameters aren't set high enough. But I also suspect that there are some people who for some reason are simply not amenable to laser hair removal.

It's important to stop using retinoids or glycolic acids three to five days before any laser (or chemical peel) treatment. They make the epidermis thinner and more vulnerable to irritation and may prevent proper healing. And because inflamed skin after being treated with laser is more prone to sunburn and postinflammatory hyperpigmentation, it's more important than ever to wear sunscreen.

the problem: Varicose and Spider Veins on Legs

WHAT A DOCTOR CALLS THEM: venulectasias (the tiny vessels on the legs)

WHAT ARE THEY?
Spider veins and varicose veins are all part of the same vascular tree of blood vessels and arteries. Varicose are the bigger, tortuous blue vessels. The smaller offshoots are fine venules, and unfortunately these can be a harbinger of possible underlying varicose veins.

WHY DO THEY HAPPEN?
This is a circulation problem stemming from incompetent valves in the vessels. These valves are supposed to prevent the backflow of blood, helping it move back up toward the brain—no easy feat considering the distance from your legs to your head and the downward pull of gravity. When they're working properly, the valves prevent blood from rushing down to the feet (another brilliant engineering facet of the body). People with varicose veins have "floppy valves" that don't open and close effectively, which causes blood to flood these leg vessels. The condition definitely worsens in pregnancy, perhaps because the blood flow doubles at that time.

This circulatory condition is partially genetic, but it can occur as a result of physical trauma too. I got my spider veins and varicose veins after a bad bicycle accident compressed my leg. In my situation, I think genetics has played a part too, and my varicose veins did get worse during my pregnancies.

HOW CAN I PREVENT THEM?
Muscle movement during exercise assists the circulation by squeezing the blood upward. So a regular exercise program—whether it's walking, running, swimming, or biking—will help greatly. Standing in one place for long periods of time can increase the risk of developing the condition

if you are already predisposed. So if you work at a job where you're on your feet for hours, you could be at risk. And yes, crossing your legs constantly may increase spider veins too, as it compresses the vessels and causes engorgement in the lower leg. I try really hard not to cross my legs when I sit down, and I have to remind myself of it all the time.

HOW CAN I TREAT THEM AT HOME?

Sadly, there are no effective do-it-yourself treatments or topical potions that will diminish the appearance of varicose or spider veins that are already present. Elevating your legs when you're at home can help, but it's no antidote. Wearing support socks or stockings can help as well.

WHAT CAN A DOCTOR DO?

First I have the patient see a radiologist or a vascular surgeon for an ultrasound test of the deeper vascular system, to see if larger vessels may have insufficient valves that could be causing the smaller spider veins. Those tiny leg veins can be treated with the same pulsed dye laser that eliminates the ones on the face. But the results on the leg are unpredictable, and many times the veins are too large for a laser to be used safely, so the best solution is a combination of laser and sclerotherapy. Sclerotherapy, injection of a saline or detergent solution, works much better on larger, more visible vessels. I use the laser as a cleanup to get rid of smaller, more superficial veins that a needle can't get into. The salt solution injected directly into the vessel is a sclerosant, a detergent that basically kills the cells. When I inject this solution, I can actually see it go up the vein, making it vasoconstrict and then disappear. As creepy as an injection of salt water or detergent into a vein sounds, it's not insanely painful. I'd say, on a scale of 1 to 10, this is a 5. The patient cannot receive a topical anesthetic because that causes vasoconstriction and makes it difficult to see the vessel. Afterward, the patient wears a compression stocking for up to seven days and should not exercise for a week. Postinflammatory hyperpigmentation due to hemosiderin (iron in the blood that's broken down) also occurs. This looks like intense bruising and can last for months (mine lasted for almost a year). I developed another side effect called "netting," where a fine network of superficial veins, almost like a fish net, showed up. (Unfortunately, this does not go away without treatment.) A patient often requires up to five treatments, and angiogenesis will keep happening over time, so veins will form again. I tell patients to expect a 50 to 90 percent improvement. If the veins are totally erased, you are lucky.

Sclerotherapy is not used to treat varicose veins, simply because the vessels are too big; injecting that much salt could ulcerate the leg. In the old days before laser surgery (as recently as ten years ago), vascular surgery was the only treatment available for varicose veins. It entails literally cutting down the leg and stripping the vein out. Severe varicose veins can be such a health hazard that they must be removed. They can lead to edema, infections, and even gangrene.

Endovenous ablation has now become a mainstream procedure, and an effective (and less invasive way) to treat the problem. I've had it done, and I can vouch for the fact that it was incredibly painful. First tumescent anesthesia (diluted lidocaine) is injected into the leg. Then a tiny incision is made and the doctor uses an ultrasound machine to guide a laser catheter through the vessel and push it all the way up through the length of the vein. As this thin cable is slowly withdrawn, the laser is fired, essentially frying the vein from within, and the vein collapses. The vein is then resorbed into the body. Thankfully, this needs to be done only once, although there are occasions when a second laser treatment is required for any vessels that remain patent, or open. Side effects can include blood clotting and thrombosis because you are heating the blood so it will congeal. (I had a clot that had to be surgically removed. Not fun.) Sounds a little like torture, right? For someone who has these ugly purple veins, it's worth the ordeal to have them treated. Nothing camouflages them, including self-tanner. I was too self-conscious to wear shorts or shorter skirts on the hottest summer day. I'm so happy with the results I've had that I would do it all again. But next time I'd do it with Valium.

>>> A REAL PATIENT STORY:
Warts and All

Warts. Even the word has a somewhat funny and embarrassing sound to it. It makes most people think of witches or toads. It's an ugly growth that can pop up on a finger or a toe. But warts can be a painful and truly debilitating medical problem. Caused by the human papillomavirus (HPV, the same family of virus that causes cervical cancer), warts can be extremely contagious and very difficult to treat. Most often they grow on hands and feet, elbows and knees—possibly because these areas are more exposed to surfaces where the virus exists. (For example, kids fall down and scrape their knees and elbows all the time, and frequently display warts there because HPV was on the ground.)

Unlike a callus—which is dead, hardened layers of skin—a wart is full of blood vessels and the HPV virus inside the cells. There are more than fifty different kinds of warts. A plantar wart (verruca plantaris) shows up on the sole of the foot ("plantar" means "foot"), and walking around barefoot can be all it takes to catch it. The wart virus is every-where—on the floor of showers and especially in public places such as the gym. A good place to catch the virus is from a rented yoga mat, so it pays to own your own. Some people are more susceptible than others (those who are ill or immunosuppressed get warts all the time). Warts are common and contagious, and in some cases they can be incapacitating.

One of my patients brought her husband to see me because he had been suffering from a horrible case of mosaic plantar warts for years. They are called "mosaic" because the bottoms of the feet are clustered with them, like cobblestone or ceramic tile. This man was a runner who had had to curtail almost all activity because even stand-ing was painful. Understandably, he became very inhibited about going barefoot in public, and he and his wife stopped spending sum-mers at the beach. He had seen other dermatologists and podiatrists and had gone through almost every conceivable treatment: liquid ni-trogen to freeze them off (a standard treatment for warts) and immu-notherapy creams such as imiquimod (the same therapy used to treat actinic keratoses and SCC precancers), which work to accelerate the

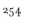

body's own attack on the area. Doctors had even tried duct tape (sometimes used to suffocate warts), and he had endured multiple surgeries to remove them. They had come back full force every single time.

I used a vascular beam laser (Vbeam, a pulsed dye laser), which targets blood vessels with a specific wavelength of light. This literally starves the wart and hopefully gets rid of it for good. The results can be excellent, but the procedure itself is expensive and extraordinarily painful. I apply numbing cream to the area first, but because the laser is literally blowing up blood vessels under the skin, it's still ten minutes of torture. After the treatment, the skin in that area becomes deeply bruised because the blood that was contained in those vessels extravasates, or travels, into the surrounding skin tissue. After the bruising, some of the warts scab and peel off, and some recede and disappear. It takes about two weeks of recovery, and the patient usually needs to have at least one to fifteen more follow-up laser treatments. Thankfully, with only two treatments, this man's warts went away completely. They haven't come back, and he and his wife just spent a happy summer at their beach house—in bare feet.

part three

>>> # REGAINING YOUR YOUTHFUL SKIN

9

Cracking the Code on Cosmeceuticals: Can Antiaging Products Make Us Look Younger, and Which Ones Really Work?

Aging. It's not a four-letter word, but it might as well be for millions of women. Growing older is inevitable, of course, but can't *looking* older be avoided—or at least delayed? As the poet Dylan Thomas wrote, "Do not go gentle into that dark night. Rage, rage against the dying of the light." Of course, the renowned poet was referring to the fierce fight against old age and death, not to women and beauty—yet his words are apt. In our youth-focused generation, aging gracefully has become oxymoronic.

Forty is now considered the new thirty, and sixty looks more like fifty thanks to ingenious scientific advances that help us look younger and younger as we get older and older. People in their forties on up aren't going to sit idly by and feel or look old if they can help it, and those in their thirties (and some in their twenties!) want to prevent it too. Pushing the boundaries of modern medicine and science has heightened our life expectancy to about 77.8 years, and now the goal is to look as young as we feel. According to a recent survey conducted by the Boomer Project, a marketing research company, female boomers feel twelve years younger than their chronological age. If there's a cure for aging, this generation of people in their forties through their sixties will surely try to find it. It's easy to argue that this is pure vanity, but I look at it as optimism. Feeling good about how you look develops a sense of confidence that is positive and productive.

It comes as no surprise, then, that sales of antiaging products in the multibillion-dollar skin care market are skyrocketing. In 2007, sales of antiaging skin care products in the United States were $1.6 billion, according to the market research firm Mintel International Group. The market grew by 63 percent from 2002 to 2007. According to another research tracking firm, the NPD Group, 60 percent of prestige skin care sales were spent on facial products that tout antiaging benefits. Antiaging is indeed big business.

I have many patients who spend hundreds, sometimes thousands, of dollars on night creams, serums, and potions containing the latest high-tech ingredients and miracle antioxidants. I imagine their medicine cabinets look like the inside of a Sephora store! All these purchases are made with the hope and desire that the products will provide dewy, fresh, youthful skin. I too understand the excitement of buying a new cream, putting it on before bed, and waking up in the morning with the anticipation that my complexion has been transformed overnight into radiant, airbrushed perfection. It's not a big challenge for cosmetic companies to romance their products and sell us a story of hope. We all want to believe that we can put something on our face that will really do what it guarantees—minimize fine lines, even out skin tone, or smooth the texture of the skin—even if these things may not be scientifically possible.

When I walk onto the beauty floor in a department store, within minutes I'm sucked into a whirlwind of pressure. It's almost like being in a Las Vegas casino—bright lights are flashing, and the whole environment is overwhelming. This promise and that promise, this cream with pomegranate extract and that lotion with some scientific-sounding ingredient, this one will take care of brown spots and that one can fix fine lines—and in just twenty-four hours. Is the $32 product as good as the one for $100? I quickly become completely confused. And I'm a dermatologist! Do these beauty counter sales-people know something I don't? This is when, to me, shopping for skin care becomes a negative experience—confounding and intimidating. I want to take that feeling out of the equation and replace it with some healthy skepticism and concrete understanding of the skin and of cosmeceuticals. If we can better understand the ingredients in these products and what they may actually be able to achieve, we can become smarter, more satisfied consumers.

Cosmeceutical Claims: Science and Pseudoscience

What is a "cosmeceutical"? Dr. Albert Kligman—the man who discovered topical retinoic acid as a treatment for acne and then wrinkles—coined the term in 1980. The word itself combines "cosmetic" and "pharmaceutical," although there's no medication to be found in the products. A cosmeceutical is a hybrid of a beauty product and an active ingredient (or a few) that may have an effect on the skin. That active element—whether it is a peptide, an antioxidant, or a growth factor—is *not* a drug, something the Food and Drug Administration considers to be anything that "affects the structure or function of the body." Only drugs are regulated (and must undergo documented clinical testing), and if they are included in a product (such as sunscreens or deodorants, for example), the label must clearly list them as active ingredients above the cosmetic ones.

As defined by the FDA, cosmetics are "articles applied to the human body for cleansing, beautifying, promoting attractiveness or altering the appearance," and they comply with only the most liberal of guidelines. Beauty products (cosmeceuticals fall under this classification) don't have to provide evidence of their efficacy, and they aren't required to undergo approval before they are sold to the public. Legally, cosmetics manufacturers don't even need to prove that their products do what they promise.

The following adjectives are incorporated into the names of some popular antiaging products: firming, lifting, renewing, detoxifying, regenerating, repairing, line-reducing, skin-transforming. When I read these labels or beauty articles that explain how a cosmeceutical can reprogram cellular division, repair DNA, or extend the life span of cells, I have to wonder. Think about it: if these ingredients really did what they promise—namely, interact with cell function and the structure of the skin—they would certainly be considered drugs and thus be regulated by the FDA. If indeed some of these chemicals fundamentally impact the skin function in a significant way (rather than just the superficial appearance), we need to validate their safety as pharmaceuticals, with stronger FDA scrutiny.

The distinction between a drug and a cosmetic is very much based on what it claims to do. If a product advertises that it eliminates wrinkles or strengthens skin cells, then it must alter the structure of the skin somehow, and therefore it must legally be considered a drug. That's one reason why most ads and labels phrase things vaguely, for instance, "minimizes the appearance of fine lines" or "gives the appearance of younger-looking skin." It's a game of white lies, since a company isn't exactly fibbing when it suggests that its product can make the skin look younger. Applying any moisturizer at all will give your skin a more youthful, less dry appearance.

For the most part, cosmetic companies do *not* back up their product claims with scientifically sound studies, and they don't have to make their research available to the public. Manufacturers usually fund experiments themselves, so it's no wonder they end up claiming positive effects. Large cosmetics companies have hundreds of cosmetic chemists and microbiologists on staff at their laboratories. *International Business News* reported that Procter & Gamble nearly doubled its beauty research staff to two thousand in the last seven years. In-house studies usually end up supporting the company's own claims, but they lack the controlled scientific methods and standards that doctors and scientists stand by. They are far from independent and objective, and the results are almost always biased. Most often, these lab studies are done in vitro, or in a test tube, not on living tissue (the in vivo method). Though an ingredient can be potent and effective in a Petri dish, that doesn't mean it will work when it's put on your skin. Who knows how it will perform when it's combined with other inactive ingredients in a delivery system such as a cream or lotion. It might be destabilized or weakened in concentration. And in vitro testing obviously does not take into consideration the obstacle of the stratum corneum. The hundred-billion-dollar question remains: Can the ingredient actually penetrate the skin to do what it claims?

The gold-standard in vitro test used to assess an ingredient's absorption through the skin is the Franz diffusion method. Scientists worldwide (including the ones at big beauty companies) utilize this technique all the time. I spoke at length with the inventor himself, Dr. Thomas Franz, who explained how his device works to measure the permeation of an ingredient. An assay (donor skin harvested from cadavers or animal tissue) is stretched across a water bath; then a medication or chemical solution is placed on the skin surface. The water in the chamber below is tested at specific time increments to gauge the percentage of chemical that has penetrated through the tissue into the reservoir. The limitation of this method is that the skin assay is not living, so it's impossible to see how an ingredient would react on the real thing. The electrical charges and chemical reactions of dynamic tissue are not in play because living cells are not functioning and their innate defense mechanisms aren't in action. It's an important test of the structural barrier of the skin, but the functional barrier of living tissue doesn't come into the picture. Dr. Franz himself emphasizes the fact that in vivo tests are very different from in vitro experiments. He has concluded that most topical ingredients don't move past the stratum corneum, although he does acknowledge that the accumulation of a chemical element on top of the skin over time (perhaps a matter of days or weeks) may increase the likelihood of its permeation.

Cosmetic researchers also use an in vivo test called skin topography analysis. This employs silicon imprints of the skin to measure wrinkle depth before and after applying a product. A gelatinous slab of silicon is pressed onto an area of skin before using a product; then a separate sheet tests the area after the product has been on the skin for various time increments (after one hour, one day, then one week). The silicon impressions are compared and the depth of the wrinkles is analyzed. This is an old technology but commonly used today because it's a safe test on human skin—even though it doesn't prove much. If the silicon sheet shows that there are fewer lines on the skin's surface (translation: "reduces the appearance of fine lines"), it is actually because crevices are being filled in by the product itself, rather than the ingredients' effecting a real change in the dermis. Other in vivo experiments use tape stripping (repeatedly ripping off tape from the surface layers of skin) to test how much of an ingredient absorbed into the stratum corneum. As interesting as the findings might be, these tests don't go deep enough, literally, to provide the scientific findings that a skin biopsy might reveal.

Because results and data are proprietary, we have no idea how most of these experiments were conducted. I've tried to get information on in-house studies a number of times and have been denied access at almost every turn. (The fine print on cosmetic advertisements sometimes offers interesting and enlightening insight, however. One ad acknowledges that its in vitro testing was done on peptides and collagen in *plants*. This is quite a few steps removed from living, human tissue.) Though true scientific research is peer-reviewed and published, studies on cosmeceuticals are usually hidden. Real science uses a double-blind study (the scientist evaluating the product doesn't know which is a placebo and which is the active ingredient) that proves the analysis is fair. Cosmeceuticals often pretend to be true science and feed us a lot of convincing-sounding scientific language in their marketing, but they're actually the antithesis. When you see "clinically proven" or "studies show" on a label, please take it with a grain of salt and read between the lines—even read the fine print in advertisements.

It's smart to question magazine articles (even doctors' quotes), advertisements, and the not-so-fine print on product labels. It's very common for dermatologists to serve as spokespeople and sit on advisory boards of cosmetic companies, lending medical credibility to a beauty product or firm. Physicians are often paid to be consultants for companies, and some conduct research for them. Most doctors will not endorse false product claims, but the wording of those claims may be vague and wishy-washy (incorporating conditional words such as "may," "can," "might," to describe what a product could possibly accomplish—with a degree of uncertainty that provides a safety net for the FDA). Be wise, and temper your expectations. Be realistic, and do your own research before purchasing a product that promises the moon. There are tons of hyped products out there making lots of money based on zero science. Educating yourself will help you take control of your beautiful skin (and your wallet). Just because a product has a made-up high-tech ingredient or an equally fictional French-sounding name doesn't make it authentically either one.

For More Information

Here are a few of my favorite Web sites that keep me informed and help me separate fact from fiction:

PubMed: www.pubmed.org: A service of the National Library of Medicine and the National Institutes of Health; this is number one for leading you to real scientific studies on specific ingredients

Environmental Working Group: www.ewg.org

www.smartskincare.com

Paula's Choice: www.cosmeticscop.com

www.ellenmarmur.com

How Skin Ages

Webster's dictionary defines senescence as "the state or process of being or becoming old." Basically our own state of senescence, or decay, involves making less of everything and slowing production down. The factory workers in the skin are heading into retirement, and their work is getting sluggish. Keratinocytes aren't turning over as fast as before, so the complexion looks dull since dead cells aren't shedding. Some studies claim that by the age of forty, the twenty-eight-day skin turnover cycle slows to forty days! There aren't as many fibroblasts replenishing themselves, and the ones that are working aren't producing collagen as plentifully.

Collagen, elastin, and chains of sugar molecules called glycosaminoglycans (GAGs), which hold water like sponges, make up the extracellular matrix in the dermis. This matrix plumps and cushions the skin like packing foam, but UV exposure and toxic oxygen radicals dissolve it every single day. The skin sags because there's less of this supportive matrix and less fat, and much of what's left is no longer firmly anchored by collagen and elastin. The epidermis becomes thinner, and there are fewer lipids and ceramides (the mortar of the stratum corneum), so the skin's barrier is drier and compromised. (The loss of estrogen at menopause exacerbates this.) Intrinsic factors (genetics, gravity, and senescence) and extrinsic factors (sun exposure, smoking, pollution, and environmental influences) intensify the negative effects of the aging process. Depressed? It's no wonder we want to believe that a skin care product can alleviate and improve this unstoppable phenomenon of getting older. Read on.

How Cosmeceuticals Promise to Work

To fight the signs of the aging process, cosmeceuticals try to prevent more degradation from happening or encourage and stimulate the senescent skin factory in the dermis to get moving. Antioxidants quench toxic free radicals, stopping them from wreaking havoc and causing inflammation, DNA mutations, and collagen destruction. Other cosmeceutical components—peptides, retinol, and growth factors, among others—are supposed to do things such as fire up collagen production, stop its destruction, slow down the aging process of skin cells, firm the skin, and increase hydration in the extracellular matrix of the dermis.

Cosmetic chemists constantly look for inspired ways to fix a problem, whether it's brown spots or wrinkles, and what they come up with makes a lot of theoretical—if not practical—sense. But the distance between theory and practice (actually putting this chemical onto your skin to get a specific result) requires a pretty giant leap in logic. For example, ingredients called peptides are either synthetically constructed or plant-derived amino acid chains that are part of a protein. This structure is similar to a protein in the body called procollagen, a precursor of collagen. When cosmetic chemists add these peptides to a Petri dish of fibroblasts, they seem to get collagen to grow in the dish. It's a brilliant discovery—in a laboratory. Many cosmeceutical ingredients replicate a substance that diminishes *inside* our bodies as we age, aiming to replace it *externally* by way of a topical product. The question comes back to how concentrated or stable the ingredient is in the delivery system and if it can penetrate through the stratum corneum to get down to the fibroblasts in the dermis. When clever advertisements and labels proclaim that a product "penetrates deep into the skin's sur-

face layers," realize what that really means: it's like a nail being hammered through surface layers of paint but not going into the wall.

The marketing of cosmeceutical ingredients and products is equally ingenious. Not only are "new discoveries" of ingredients being developed, but cosmetic companies come up with new (and almost scientifically plausible) skin problems to fix too. In chapter 3, I discussed glycation (the process by which carbohydrates and sugars we ingest in our diet may attach to proteins like collagen inside the body and degrade them). New skin care products have been created in an attempt to remedy this glycation problem, but there are no human-controlled studies on how glycation affects the skin or on the effectiveness of cosmeceutical fixes. Do we need a product that may or may not penetrate the surface of the skin to counteract a problem that may or may not have anything to do with the skin?

Believe me, I love to buy this stuff just as much as you do, but I resent the fact that I'm being manipulated into thinking that a skin care product is doing more than it possibly can. The fact is that these topical ingredients are probably not going far enough through the surface of the skin to make any significant changes to collagen production or anything else in the dermis. They do, however, have a wonderful superficial effect, although it is temporary. Any good moisturizer is going to minimize wrinkles and immediately make the skin look fresher and appear more youthful. And many antiaging products include ingredients that offer a kind of optical illusion. Silicone is used to smooth and "fill in" fine lines, while silica or polymers in a firming product either tighten the top of the skin or leave a stiff film on the surface. Many expensive antiaging creams and lotions contain light-diffusing ingredients such as mica or even micronized diamond particles (now, that makes for a pricey face cream!) that refract light and blur the appearance of wrinkles. The same elements are used in makeup to magically improve the complexion. They manipulate the appearance of the top layer of skin, and they work—but it all washes off with water.

The Laws of Penetration and Absorption:
How Topical Ingredients Can Get Through Our Gore-tex

Do you recall how I promised that reading chapter 1, the explanation of the architecture of the skin, would be important? Well, here's why. Let's go back to what is contained in the dermis: collagen and elastin, all the spongy foam (the GAGs) of the extracellular matrix, blood vessels, nerves, and sweat and oil glands. And remember that above this layer is the cement level of the basement membrane that is glued to the dermis, the brick wall of the stratum granulosem and the Gore-tex of the stratum corneum. The epidermis is a formidable barrier that keeps good things in the skin and bad things out. It is obviously tough, if not nearly impossible, to bypass it. So if a product claims to stimulate collagen, for instance, it has to get down to the dermis, where the collagen and fibroblasts are. But do these ingredients ever get there? Let's look at how it can be done.

Once you put a cream or lotion on your face, what happens? When it sits on top of your skin, the complexion appears hydrated, smoother, and healthier. But do those miracle ingredients ever make the journey down to the extracellular matrix? There are two ways any topical ingredient can get through the skin: either by penetrating the bricks and mortar (the skin cells and fatty ceramides) of the intact epidermis or by taking a hypothetical shortcut through the pores (the follicles and sweat glands). The pores allow ingredients to bypass the first stratum corneum layer and go farther down, where they have a better chance of getting into the dermis. But the walls of the tunnel-like follicle still have the bricks-and-mortar structure and basement membrane surrounding it, so the obstacles and locked doors to the dermis still exist. It would probably easier for you or me to get into the Pentagon than for a chemical to get into the skin. But it is *not* impossible. If an ingredient meets most of the following important criteria, it has a fighting chance of reaching its destination.

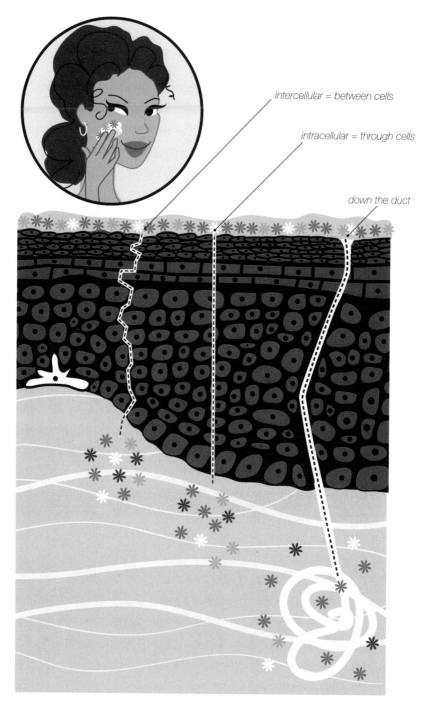

The three pathways of skin penetration when you apply a product

Four Characteristics That Allow an Ingredient to Penetrate Through the Skin

The Small Size of the Ingredient's Molecules

An ingredient must be tiny enough to get through the epidermis or the pores. For example, the collagen molecule is far too large to penetrate past the surface of the skin. It can only sit on top. This is why nanotechnology (a nanometer is a billionth of a meter) and microencapsulation are hot topics in the cosmetic world right now. Chemists are shrinking ingredient particles to a microscopic molecular weight in order for them to permeate the cell membrane that has microscopic channels that might allow a microsized particle through. (Nanotechnology is also being used with zinc oxide and titanium dioxide in sunscreens to make the formulations more transparent.) Besides nanosizing ingredients, they can be suspended in microscopic silica shells that may possibly be able to penetrate the epidermis. Ideally, once the microsphere reaches the dermis it will go through a chemical reaction that disintegrates the capsule and releases the ingredient inside, allowing it to be absorbed. One prescription retinoid uses microsphere technology to better penetrate the skin without causing as much irritation as usual. These kinds of formulation enhancements are the wave of the future for cosmeceuticals, creating James Bond-like molecules that can go anywhere and do anything.

The Ingredient's Chemical Compatibility with the Skin

Basic chemistry teaches us that like substances are compatible. In the case of a chemical ingredient, its positive or negative energy charge, its pH balance, and its temperature must all be in harmony with the skin in order to permeate it. The acid mantle on the skin's surface, a fine film containing sweat, sebum, and amino acids, is yet another barrier that protects the skin from infection. If an ingredient is compatible with the skin's own pH (which is around 5.7), it has a better chance to slip under the radar rather than irritate the skin. Ingredients that alter the delicate pH balance too much are harsh and will destroy skin cells. Alpha-hydroxy acids, for example, are so acidic that they eat through the surface of the skin, generating a chemical exfoliation of the stratum corneum that's ultimately beneficial. The positive or negative electrical charge of an ion also assists in pushing it through the skin, while the lack of a compatible magnetic force won't allow a material to stick. This is similar to trying to attach the wrong side of a magnet to a re-frigerator—the magnet just slips off. The temperature of a product and how it's influenced by body temperature will also affect how it blends into the skin. Like putting a pat of cold butter on an untoasted piece of bread, temperature incompatibility won't allow it to melt in—it can only sit on the surface.

The Ingredient's Water or Fat Solubility

The stratum corneum is packed tight with skin cells (bricks) and fatty lipids (mortar), so to move through this tier an ingredient must be compatible with one of them. Theoretically, lipophilic, or fatty, mole-cules can penetrate fat easily—taking an intercellular approach mean-ing that they move in between the cells through the fatty lipids (mortar). Aquaphilic, or water-soluble, ingredients may be able to pass through watery cells, taking a transcellular path. But each cell has its own individual barrier, the fatty cell membrane, which makes infiltra-tion tricky. An ingredient has to be watery but moderately lipophilic too. Cosmetic chemists add enhancers, chemicals that make a mole-cule more compatible and thus make an ingredient more permeable. The addition of a fat molecule, for example, could make a watery in-gredient just lipophilic enough to pass through the cell membrane and move on to the dermis.

The Ingredient's Stability

It is common for a chemical to become unstable when exposed to light or oxygen in air and thereby lose its effectiveness. Vitamin C, a strong antioxidant, is notoriously difficult to keep stable in its topical form. Once it is exposed to oxygen, it's deactivated and may even become irritating to the skin. The chemist's challenge is to make sure the active ingredient remains stable and effective both inside a product's container and out.

An ingredient can also become ineffective simply by being applied it the wrong way. Again using vitamin C as an example, if it is applied to damp skin it becomes destabilized and inactivated. Putting one product over another can also decrease the chance of absorption, so putting a retinoid or another active ingredient onto clean skin increases its chances of breaking through the stratum corneum. Completely dry skin can be another barrier to ingredients. Applying a lipophilic or aquaphilic product onto a dried-out surface is like putting a cream or lotion on a stone—it just sits there or slides off because there are no pathways in which to move deeper. Water- or fat-soluble ingredients need a hydrated surface to travel through. See? This is tricky stuff.

Delivery Systems: Enhancing the Potential for Permeation

After most of these four problems are solved, what methods of application might improve an ingredient's potential for absorption? Supersaturation (using excessive amounts of a product on the skin) helps guarantee that enough active ingredient might get through the epidermis. (It's an impractical and expensive solution when it comes to skin care products, I admit.) It is more likely that a cosmeceutical that's used regularly over days and weeks will accumulate either on the skin or in the pores. If it doesn't wash off when it saturates the follicles or the glands, the residual might eventually penetrate into the dermis. It has been found with topical steroids that the cumulative application is what makes the medication effective and also conveys some risk. Nevertheless, the concentration of active ingredient is key.

Another means of penetrating the skin is occlusion and physical force—literally pushing something into the skin. Mesotherapy, for instance, utilizes injections to deliver small amounts of active ingredients or pharmaceuticals directly into the dermis. Some doctors use it to get anti-inflammatory medications right to the source for pain management. It's been employed, with less success, as a way to fight fat and cellulite with a concoction of vitamins and botanicals pumped into the dermis. In Europe (and less so in the United States), any "active" ingredients that are included in cosmeceuticals have been used in mesotherapy. It's interesting that some of the doctors who pioneered mesotherapy in the 1990s have stopped using the technique because of adverse side effects. This method of permeating the skin was never shown to work effectively, and therefore it never really took off.

There are other, less invasive techniques that can force ingredients further into the skin. Transdermal patches, like nicotine or hormone patches, use this occlusive approach to help diffuse a concentrated dose of medication or chemical through the skin and into the bloodstream. This utilizes all the methods possible for tissue penetration namely—a high concentration of medication and a penetration enhancer of occlusion to hold it on the skin.

Does this mean we'll soon be able to buy "peptide patches"? The delivery system has been proven to work for medications, and cosmetic companies have already come out with antiaging versions (although objective scientific studies have yet to vet these new products). But this method raises an important question about the negative possibilities of topical ingredients permeating the skin. If a substance can reach the dermis, it can also get into the bloodstream. Then it becomes a question of how toxic it might be or if it could be dangerous in some way. For example, if an ingredient that claims to make skin cells proliferate or change their DNA gets into the dermis (and the vascular system), it could cause cell mutations that in turn might create cancers. It's a scary thought and a case of be careful what you wish for with scientific advances. If a substance penetrates the skin successfully, don't you want it to be safety-tested as a drug by the FDA?

Antiaging Products:
Four Rules to Remember Before You Start Shopping

Some products state that they prevent and reverse the signs of aging. Others claim to firm, smooth, and lift the skin, and there are plenty that guarantee they stimulate collagen and diminish wrinkles. Antiaging products do fill our heads with promises. (I completely expect to wake up looking like Gwyneth Paltrow after using one.) There are thousands to pick from, from pricey prestige brands to drugstore options that are more reasonably priced. How can you choose between them, and which ingredients actually might work?

Most of us feel baffled and frustrated, with way too many choices. (Remember my overwhelming shopping trip?) According to the American Academy of Dermatology in Schaumburg, Illinois, 94 percent of women are confused by their antiaging options. So let's demystify the cosmeceutical mystery. There are four rules to remember:

1. Prevent aging skin with what you already own: sunscreen.

Sun protection is the best antiaging product you have and the best investment you can make. Ninety percent of cosmetic skin problems that occur with age (wrinkles, sagging, hyperpigmentation) are caused by sun exposure, according to the *Journal of the American Academy of Dermatology*. Therefore sunscreen is the best honest-to-goodness miracle cream on the market. There is no point in buying a bunch of antiaging products to repair damage if you don't prevent it in the first place by wearing sunscreen every day. Most cosmeceutical ingredients try to mimic substances found in the body, such as antioxidants, peptides, growth factors, coenzymes, copper, and vitamins. So protecting what we already have naturally and maintaining optimal skin health with daily sun protection and moisturizer is worth a thousand antiaging beauty solutions. In fact, as I mentioned in chapter 4, I have a collection of sunscreens and I use them all differently—an oil-free, broad-spectrum SPF 15 for daily use; an SPF 30 when I know I'll be outside more of the day; a body lotion with added sunscreen; and an even stronger broad-spectrum sunscreen spray for the beach. Because your skin type changes and the amount of sun exposure you receive does too, your sun protection needs to be compatible. Owning several formulations of sunscreen also reduces the excuses not to wear it, and sunscreens are a better investment than a bunch of cosmeceuticals. Think about it this way: every time you put on sunscreen, you're preventing the signs of aging and therefore saving money on expensive products or cosmetic procedures to fix fine lines or sun spots.

2. Read product labels closely.

The label must list ingredients from the highest concentration to the lowest, so if the antiaging element you're looking for, be it niacinamide or vitamin C, is near the bottom, there's not enough in the product to do anything. (Keep in mind; a high concentration of the chemical is one way to get it into the skin). Most often, a cosmeceutical acts primarily as a good moisturizer, which is wonderful, but it won't have much more than superficial and temporary results. Most of the ingredients on the label—the water, moisturizers, binders, and preservatives that make up the vehicle (see chapter 4)—are inactive. Often an antiaging product includes silicone to provide a smooth texture to the product and make the complexion look smoother too. It may also contain a little glycolic acid or lactic acid to exfoliate the skin and provide instant gratification. These elements don't actually change anything below the surface of your skin. At least make sure that the antioxidant or peptide you're buying is very near the top of the ingredients list. Decoding the label has limitations, however. Most of the time a product does not state the concentration or percentage of the ingredients (and it doesn't have to). And too high a concentration of some ingredients, such as vitamin C, can be toxic to the skin. You also can't tell from the label whether an ingredient, like an antioxidant, is stable or not.

3. Choose your antiaging ingredients wisely.

Okay, let's shift gears. Let's pretend that all these cosmeceuticals work. With so many new ingredients promising to fix so many problems, how should you decide among them? Do you need an antioxidant or a peptide? And what is a growth factor, anyway? Is a prescription retinoid safe, or should you try an over-the-counter version first? Step back, look at your skin, and consider what products you already own. A moisturizer? A sunscreen? A chemical exfoliant or a scrub? (Check to see if your moisturizer already contains an antioxidant or one of the ingredients I'll discuss soon. You may have been using an antiaging product for some time without even knowing it.) Ask yourself what you are trying to achieve with a cosmeceutical. Are you in your twenties and looking for a preventive product? An antioxidant is a good bet. Do you want to fight wrinkles? Then something with retinoic acid will work. If brown spots and uneven skin tone are your problem, you can use retinoic acid or try a product with niacinamide. Narrow down what it is about your complexion you want to improve, and that will help narrow down your options.

Tending to your complexion is like caring for a garden, which needs a certain amount of water, nutrients, soil, and sunshine to grow and be healthy. If you overfeed or overwater it, the garden is destroyed. In the same way, putting too much of a good thing on your skin is not necessarily better or more effective. I've had patients come in with red, irritated skin and show me twenty different products that they use on it. How do all these ingredients react with one another? Are they overlapping the same kinds of chemicals, such as acids, over and over again? Try to pick one or two active ingredients—an antioxidant and a retinoid, for instance—and stick with them for at least three months (a fair amount of time to see if you get results). Switching from one ingredient to another within a span of a couple of weeks—a niacinamide product, then a kojic acid, then an azeleic acid to get rid of brown spots, for example—can create a cocktail of chemicals on your face that can be extremely irritating.

4. Research products, and learn the difference between miracles and marketing.

Do your homework on ingredients, and think logically about their claims. Frequently what is proclaimed to be a new chemical innovation turns out to be a derivative of something that already exists. For instance, an exciting ingredient (whose name was created and patented by a cosmetic company) claims to stimulate the production of glycosaminoglycans (GAGs) and increase the storage of moisture in the dermis. This chemical has a cool, sci-fi name and sounds like an amazing discovery, yet it's simply a plant-derived form of xylose (a sugar molecule like the GAGs). Again, the manufacturer's tests are proprietary, and most products containing the ingredient also include hyaluronic acid, a superior humectant. So it's hard to say which one is responsible for any water retention results in the skin. A little sleuthing online can tell you what a hot new ingredient actually is and if the clinical studies behind it are for real.

Most of these ingredients aren't really under the jurisdiction of a dermatologist. Traditional medical training has nothing to do with a popular antioxidant like CoffeeBerry, or an ingredient like rare, Japanese seaweed. As a doctor, I must form a medically educated opinion about whether these things provide substantial results or not. I read the claims and the literature available, put them through my dermatologic understanding of the body, and judge if it's a reasonable hypothesis or not. So far three things have been proven to work as anti-agers: sunscreen, moisturizer (to maintain the health of the skin's barrier), and retinoic acid.

Cosmeceutical Ingredients: What Are They, and Which Ones Really Work?

Do any of these skin-transforming miracle ingredients do what they promise to? Only time and strong scientific studies will tell. Now that you are wise to how the skin works, you may not be as easily persuaded to buy a product until you get some firm facts. Go back, scan the four rules I just gave you, and ask yourself some questions: What exactly is this miracle ingredient? Is it present in a high enough concentration in this product? Is it stable in the vehicle (the cream, lotion, or serum)? Could the ingredient possibly penetrate the skin? What follows is a review of the most popular ingredients in antiaging products, their marketing claims, the facts—based on limited to no published data—and my recommendations.

KEY

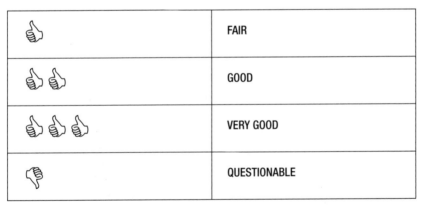

	FAIR
	GOOD
	VERY GOOD
	QUESTIONABLE

Retinoic Acid

The various forms (tretinoin, tazarotene, adapalene) available on prescription are all chemical derivatives of vitamin A. Nonprescription retinol is a weaker analog (a synthetic copy), which must be converted to retinoic acid inside the skin cells in order to work.

The Claims: Originally developed as an acne treatment by Dr. Albert Kligman in 1967, tretinoin was soon discovered to improve signs of photoaging, like wrinkles and brown spots, and help firm and smooth the skin. A true miracle antiaging drug was born, and more than twenty years later it is still the gold standard of antiaging topicals. It has been proven in numerous tests to stimulate collagen production and decrease collagen loss, which means fewer wrinkles and plumper skin over time. It regulates cell turnover, which results in less hyperpigmentation and brighter, more radiant skin (since dead cells are shed off efficiently), and decreases fine lines.

The Facts: This is one time where all the claims are factual, since this drug has been proven to penetrate to the dermis and act directly on the skin cells. Retinoic acid works by communicating with retinoid receptors on the cells and signaling chemical reactions. (Different forms of retinoic acid click on a different molecular switch, or receptor, so each produces slightly different results. This is why one type may be better for acne and another more effective for antiaging.) Once triggered, these receptors prompt cell growth and collagen and elastin synthesis. Retinoic acid regulates cell turnover and the shedding of dead cells on the surface; it builds up the extracellular matrix by stimulating collagen production and ultimately increases volume, thickness, and firmness. It repairs DNA damage in skin cells and inhibits the enzymes that break down collagen.[1] Improvement is gradual (it should be seen within a few months) but significant.

Prescription retinoids are the strongest and most effective form of retinoic acid. Over-the-counter products contain milder vitamin A analogs; either retinol or retinyl palmitate (retinyl palmitate being the weakest). In order to have an effect on retinoid receptors, these must be converted to retinoic acid inside the body, and that conversion may not happen with the trace amount of low-strength vitamin A contained in a beauty product. Although the results are therefore inconsistent, an

OTC retinol might be worth a try if you're skittish about using a prescription medication or if you have especially sensitive skin. Stabilized, high-strength retinol may be somewhat effective, but look for one that states the percentage of retinol on the label. Otherwise there's probably just a tiny, ineffectual amount in the product. (Personally, I would rather use a prescription retinoid with a percentage of medication that I know works.)

Side Effects: Retinoic acid is a drug and there are risks associated with its use. Since it decreases sebum (remember, this is still an acne medicine), it makes the skin extremely dry. (If that's the case for you, applying moisturizer on top of retinoic acid is the answer, and it won't dilute its potency.) It makes the skin photosensitive, so daily sunscreen is a must—which is also why retinoic acid should be used at night. It tends to irritate even moderately sensitive skin, so be careful not to overdo exfoliants such as glycolic acids (once a week is plenty). For the same reason, be sure to stop using retinoids three to five days before having any skin procedure done, from simple waxing and facials to medical peels or lasers. For those who have a hard time tolerating even a low-dose prescription retinoid, I recommend trying short-term applications: apply a pea-size amount over the whole face and neck, leave it on for fifteen minutes, then rinse it off. You may get the same benefits as wearing it overnight.

My Bottom Line: Retinoic acid is the only topical antiaging product that is proven to penetrate into the dermis and work on a cellular level to improve skin.

👍 👍 👍 Retin-A is the established gold standard and universally recommended for antiaging.

FORMS OF RETINOIC ACID	BRANDS	CHARACTERISTICS & FACTS
Tretinoin	Retin-A, Retin-A Micro, Renova	All use a 0.02% to 0.05% concentration of tretinoin. Renova is in a more emollient base. Retin-A Micro is encapsulated and therefore less irritating and possibly more effective.
Tazarotene	Avage, Tazorac	Is faster acting than tretinoin and can be more irritating.
Adapalene	Differin	Can be less irritating than tretinoin. Used primarily as a treatment for acne.
Retinol	OTC brands	1.0% is the strongest concentration available OTC. Most brands contain less than 0.5%.
Retinaldehyde	OTC brands	A precursor of tretinoin and less effective.
Retinyl palmitate	OTC brands	The weakest of the OTC versions.

>>> A REAL PATIENT STORY:
A Surprising Risk Factor for Retinoic Acids

A recent situation with one of my patients brings up the distressing question of cutaneous penetration of the skin and potential toxicity of topical application of retinoic acid. This forty-five-year-old woman has been using a prescription-strength retinoid three times a week for approximately a year. Since she also has osteoporosis and hormonal issues, her endocrinologist does a regular lab workup as part of a bi-annual checkup. Her last blood tests showed an extraordinarily high level of vitamin A in her system. Since this woman's diet hasn't changed at all, the logical conclusion is that the source of this overload of vitamin A may be due to the topical retinoids she is using.

Medical studies have found that excessive dietary intake of vitamin A is associated with decreased bone mineral density and increase risk of fractures.[2] In animals, retinoic acid has been shown to decrease osteoblast activity and reduce the ability of vitamin D to absorb calcium.[3]

This information brings to light significant issues that deserve further scientific investigation: Can the cumulative topical application of retinoic acid cause hypervitaminosis? If so, should women at risk of osteoporosis (many women over forty years old who are the prime users of topical retinoids) discontinue topical retinoic acid? Must they choose between younger skin and healthier bones? This patient's endocrinologist has urged her to stop using retinoids, but she's so happy with the antiaging results that she's hesitant to do so. There haven't been many documented cases of this, so don't panic. But let your doctor know about *all* chemicals you are using on your body, as well as drugs you take systemically.

Niacinamide and N-acetyl Glucosamine

Niacinamide is a derivative of vitamin B3, or niacin. Also known as nicotinic acid, this is a precursor of the energy-producing coenzymes in the body called nicotinamide adenine dinucleotides (NADs), which are consumed in all sorts of metabolic processes, including cell growth and lipid production.

N-acetyl glucosamine is a stable form of glucosamine, an amino derivative of glucose in the body that's a precursor of glycosaminoglycans (GAGs), chains of amino sugar molecules. In the skin GAGs hold water like sponges to cushion and protect the skin.

The Claims: These two ingredients are usually combined into a complex, holding on to each other in order to work better together. They reduce brown spots by allegedly slowing down melanin production, and niacinamide is supposed to block melanosomes from reaching the epidermis. They are excellent humectants, since N-acetyl glucosamine is a component of the GAGs that bind water in the skin. Niacinamide has also been found to rev up the skin's production of ceramides.

The Facts: Both ingredients have been proven to be stable and safe, and there are some decent data to support their claims. A placebo-controlled, double-blind in vivo study involving more than two hundred subjects reported that topical niacinamide and N-acetyl glucosamine, when paired in a formulation, significantly reduced the appearance of hyperpigmented skin.[4] In vitro studies have proven that the ingredients stimulate hyaluronan synthesis.[5]

My Bottom Line: If your main issue is brown spots, it wouldn't hurt to give a product containing niacinamide and N-acetyl glucosamine a try. The added benefit of hydrating the skin is a gift with purchase. Some valid science backs up both those assertions. It's important to understand that the concentration of ingredients in an over-the-counter product is unknown, so it is unclear whether you will get enough of either to make much of a change in your complexion.

👍 It could be promising and worth trying.

Antioxidants

This is a huge category, and under this umbrella are vitamins (such as C and E), botanical extracts containing powerful antioxidant compounds called polyphenols (green tea, CoffeeBerry, pomegranate, and resveratrol from grapes). The term also includes natural fatty acids such as alpha-lipoic acid and synthetic antioxidants such as idebenone, an analog (synthetic impersonator) of coenzyme Q10, a natural antioxidant present in our cells that produces energy. Plant nutrients such as flavonoids (present in soy and wild yam) are considered potent antioxidant and anti-inflammatory agents as well.

The Claims: A remedy for sun damage and the free radicals that are generated by it, antioxidants neutralize those free radicals and work as anti-inflammatories. In this way, they indirectly stop deterioration of collagen and damage to DNA in skin cells and consequently prevent new wrinkles from forming. Many antioxidants, whether applied topically or taken orally, have been found to enhance sun protection, although they are no substitute for sunscreen. Antioxidants brighten the skin by controlling the destructive toxic radical cascade that ultimately leaves dead, dull cells on the surface. Some, like vitamin C, have been proven to actually build collagen (vitamin C is a cofactor, an essential component, in collagen synthesis).

The Facts: Antioxidants are practically billed as cure-alls, and a new, improved form pops up every few months. (The latest botanical wonders are acai berry and phloretin from apples.) Antioxidants are definitely not overnight fixes, and it might take time for them to work. *Directly,* antioxidants may preserve the normal function of the skin and prevent toxic radicals from killing cells and collagen off too soon. *Indirectly,* this leads to skin brightening and diminishing of pigmentation and fine lines. They help to avert UV damage and have an anti-inflammatory effect, which consequently slows the breakdown of collagen. But with almost every one of these ingredients, the biggest obstacle to efficacy is stability.

Vitamin C has been proven to be a strong antioxidant. It's also been found to stimulate collagen production and perhaps to inhibit MMPs too. Remember, citric acid is a natural alpha-hydroxy exfoliant, which will slough off brown spots and dull skin. Unfortunately, the instability factor is a big catch. There are quite a few forms of the vitamin (L-ascorbic acid, ascorbyl palmitate, and others), but the instability of all these forms is what makes effective topical use tricky. Though L-ascorbic acid might be stable in a laboratory, by the time it gets onto your skin it can oxidize and become inactive. In fact, oxidized vitamin C may actually cause free-radical formation. Often, products include vitamin E to back up ascorbic acid's antioxidant effects, just in case

they are degraded. These two vitamins work synergistically, multiply-
ing their positive effects when they are used together. Look for a product that contains around 10% vitamin C (less won't be effective); it
should be in an opaque container that doesn't let in light. Note that
more than 10% concentration can actually create more free radicals by
stimulating chemical reactions in the skin. Unfortunately, since the
percentages are often left off of OTC labels, it's impossible to tell how
much is contained in a product.

Polyphenols, potent antioxidant compounds found in green tea,
pomegranate, resveratrol, and the new CoffeeBerry, are currently the
most popular kids in the antioxidant class. Studies have shown that
topical caffeine from green and black teas repairs UV damage, and
the active polyphenols provide strong antioxidant, anti-inflammatory, and anticarcinogenic benefits.[6] Most cosmeceuticals, however,
don't contain a high enough concentration of polyphenols, and certainly not the high levels that drinking brewed green tea would
supply. (If a cosmetic contains the 5% green tea extract necessary to
be effective topically, the product should be brown.) Again, the big
problem is instability.

Resveratrol, a polyphenol compound found in the skin of red
grapes, is being studied for its ability to activate enzymes in the body
called sirtuins, which help extend the life span of cells. Sirtuins kick in
as a natural response to the need for tissue preservation. This response
is the body's survival mechanism to keep cells alive longer in case of
starvation. A recent study found that the life spans of mice dosed with
large amounts of resveratrol were extended by 30 percent.[7] This dem-
onstrates the sometimes humorous comparison of scientific theory to
practice: to get similar results from resveratrol, humans would have to
consume about thirty-five bottles of red wine a day! Resveratrol is also
being tested for its antioxidant and anti-inflammatory properties, although the results have been contradictory. One study in mice showed
that it reduced free-radical damage by UV light,[8] but an in vitro experiment found that the presence of resveratrol increased DNA mutations

in skin cell cultures when exposed to UVA light.[9] All this goes to show that more research needs to be conducted.

The antioxidant compound in CoffeeBerry is extracted from the unripe fruit of the coffee plant (the beans are actually pits). It also contains polyhydroxy acid, which exfoliates the skin and has a brightening effect. This antioxidant is relatively new on the scene, and so far the company that developed and manufactures it has sponsored the only clinical tests. Though CoffeeBerry may be as powerful as it sounds, I'm curious to read more about scientific studies done in the future; I hope they will be made available to the public.

Clinical studies can be confusing to decipher. Idebenone, for example, was found in one study to have stronger oxidative stress protection capacity than vitamin C (L-ascorbic acid), vitamin E (tocopherol), or alpha-lipoic acid.[10] But other studies have refuted that finding.[11] Another study did skin biopsies on a small number of patients who used idebenone and found that they had decreased levels of MMPs and an increase in collagen.[12]

So which antioxidant should you choose? The news is encouraging for all of them, but stability and concentration vary among products. Again, doing your homework is key, but it's not easy. I think almost all of these antioxidants hold promise, but it's too soon to say for the majority of them. Most existing studies are pretty small, in vitro, or biased, and the available literature is limited and somewhat confusing.

My Bottom Line: I have discussed the power of antioxidants in a healthy diet, as a protective force against sun damage, as possible cancer fighters, and as superheroes battling the toxic free radicals that damage DNA in cells. It is a convincing argument that a potent, stable, concentrated form of a topical antioxidant could also be effective from the outside in. The advice "everything in moderation" bears repeating here, and it's probable that most cosmeceuticals don't contain antioxidants that are concentrated or stable enough to be truly effective. *Eating* antioxidants, rather than putting them on your face, may provide better results. There's no proven harm in using skin care products containing antioxidants, but in order to benefit from them, try to find ones with an appropriately high concentration of stable ingredients. Try to keep the buzz and hype behind the hot new antioxidants in perspective, and check out the available research first.

👍 👍 Antioxidants can be beneficial, but choose products with the best, most stable ingredients.

Kinetin

Kinetin (N6-furfuryladenine) is a form of cytokinin, a plant-derived growth hormone that promotes cell division and slows the aging process in plant cells.

The Claim: This ingredient has antioxidant and anti-inflammatory benefits and has been hyped as a more natural, less irritating alternative to retinoic acid.

The Facts: A multitude of established scientific studies done over the last twenty years has proved retinoic acid's effect on regulating cell turnover and stimulating collagen production. In comparison, hardly any comparable research backs up the notion that kinetin works in the same way. It's a logical, yet implausible, stretch that a synthetic plant hormone that promotes cell division and retards senescence in plants could do the same thing in human skin. The two studies showing that kinetin affects cell differentiation in keratinocytes and fibroblasts were done in vitro. It has been proven to be a good antioxidant (also in vitro), and that effect may indirectly preserve collagen. Studies have not shown that kinetin causes an elongation of the life span of collagen, but an improvement of its overall health.

My Bottom Line: Kinetin is safe, well tolerated, and a decent antioxidant. It can't replace the formidable and proven results of retinoic acid, however. For someone with sensitive skin, I would advise trying short applications of a prescription retinoid. But for those who are turned off by retinoids entirely, this might be a decent alternative.

Kinetin is a fair antioxidant, but not proven to provide the same results as retinoic acid.

Epidermal Growth Factors

Epidermal growth factors (EGFs) are derived from plants or human fetal fibroblasts, or bioengineered from human skin. Growth factors communicate with cells, spurring reactions such as cell division and wound healing.

The Claim: Like kinetin, a plant growth factor, these human or bioengineered versions claim to do the same thing: slow the aging process in the skin and trigger cell proliferation. Products containing growth factors claim to diminish fine lines and brown spots and improve skin texture and elasticity.

The Facts: The body is full of various kinds of growth hormones. They act as messengers, each type binding to its respective receptor on a cell to tell it to do something. Ideally, some of the growth factors in a cream can coax fibroblasts to produce more collagen, for example. A product containing EGFs usually includes a blend of different growth factors (attained or engineered from different tissue sources). I have yet to find a strong double-blind, human-controlled study that backs up any of the interesting claims behind epidermal growth factors.

My Bottom Line: Another fascinating concept, but in practice it's questionable whether (1) the active ingredients will penetrate the skin (since growth factors are large molecules), (2) they will remain stable and effective, (3) they are concentrated enough, (4) the specific growth factors will reach their specific receptors to do their specific rejuvenation job. Almost all products containing growth factors also include antioxidants or glycolic acid to ensure some positive results, at least superficially.

Though epidermal growth factors may be safe, their topical use is questionably effective as a collagen producer.

Peptides

A peptide is an amino acid chain that forms a protein.

The Claim: Peptides, as precursors of proteins such as collagen, provide the building blocks and the stimulus for cells to produce more. These fragments of proteins act as messengers, communicating between cells. Cosmeceuticals contain engineered peptides such as palmitoyl pentapeptide-4 (trademarked as Matrixyl by corporations like Sederma and Procter & Gamble), a small molecule consisting of five linked amino acids. Palmitoyl pentapeptide-4 is attached to a fatty acid that enhances its ability to penetrate the skin (making it oil-soluble).

The Facts: Much like growth factors, peptides are a bioengineered version of a natural element in the body. (Some natural moisturizers contain plant peptides, derived from wheat or rice. Along the same lines as kinetin, which has a plant growth factor, these may work as well as biotech versions. Considering that we don't know what will penetrate the skin anyway, why not?) The idea of adding peptides to the skin is theoretically like sending in a surge of troops to carry out repair and regeneration. In vitro tests have found that pentapeptide-4 does prompt fibroblasts to produce more collagen in cell cultures. (As usual, there is a serious lack of truly objective data since the companies that manufacture the peptide ingredients have funded most of the studies.) And remember, a cell culture is a dish of cells and is a far cry from your skin.

My Bottom Line: Can peptides penetrate to the dermis to stimulate collagen production? Without scientific studies that biopsy the skin, it's difficult to assess whether they can and if they really work. The inspiration behind these ingredients makes sense, and time will tell if some may be effective antiagers. Because peptides happen to be effective humectants, a product containing them will successfully hold moisture in the skin.

👍 They're worth a try, especially since you're assured of getting an excellent humectant and most include antioxidant components too.

MMP Inhibitors (MMPIs)

Matrix metalloproteinases (MMPs) are enzymes (one of which is collagenase) that break down and eliminate old or damaged proteins such as collagen and GAGs. Inhibitors aim to slow that process and increase the retention of the cushioning in the extracellular matrix.

The Claim: MMPI ingredients (in most products these are a patented mixture of botanical elements) allegedly stop the proliferation of MMPs and their ability to scavenge collagen, elastin, and GAGs in the dermis.

The Facts: This is another cosmeceutical element that makes theoretical sense: attempting to stop the destruction of the extracellular matrix by suppressing an overload of MMPs. Retinoic acid has been proven to do this indirectly. And sunscreens and anti-inflammatory ingredients, such as antioxidants, may prevent the production of more MMPs in the first place, since less collagen is damaged. The patented MMPIs in some cosmeceuticals appear to be formulated from a blend of botanical extracts, but I'm not sure how these affect enzymes in the dermis. (I have a hunch that some of the extracts have anti-inflammatory or antioxidant properties that may work indirectly.)

My Bottom Line: As always, I question whether the ingredients in an over-the-counter product can reach the dermis to do this job, but even if they could, would we want to stop the body's natural recycling process and its disposal of inferior structural proteins? Though cosmetic companies have done proprietary in vitro tests, there are no conclusive scientific studies that prove that MMPIs permeate the skin, inhibit MMP activity, or lead to more robust collagen. Using an antioxidant in combination with retinoic acid would be a more reliable way to preserve the extracellular matrix and prevent the loss of collagen.

It's doubtful that a product containing these inhibitors will do more than moisturize the skin effectively.

Dimethylaminoethanol (DMAE)

This is an organic compound found in the body that's involved in the synthesis of neurotransmitters in the brain associated with cognitive function and muscle contraction. DMAE taken orally has been used to increase mental alertness by stimulating the release of these neurotransmitters.

The Claim: Topical skin care products containing DMAE claim that it makes skin look firmer, smoother, and less lined and that it immediately improves elasticity.

The Facts: These claims are probably partially true, but the way that DMAE works topically to instantly plump and tighten the skin is by inducing swelling of the skin cells.[13] In vitro research has discovered that the chemical has the same swelling effect on fibroblasts and that this may kill them.[14] These studies point out some serious, toxic complications (if indeed DMAE can penetrate to the dermis). They definitely provide an incentive for more research into the ingredient's safety and efficacy.

My Bottom Line: Without a doubt, almost anything is toxic in huge concentrations (even water), but these studies are noteworthy enough to encourage caution. There aren't any conclusive, objective scientific studies that I'm aware of regarding the positive effects of topical DMAE.

This ingredient has only some shaky science backing it up, and some studies have found it to be potentially dangerous.

Copper Peptides

Copper is a trace mineral in the body, essential for many biochemical processes, including metabolism—it allows numerous enzymes to function properly—and maintenance of connective tissue in the body.

The Claim: As a topical ingredient, the copper atom is tightly bound with protein peptides, creating a compound. In 1993, it was discovered to be effective in healing wounds and reducing scar tissue (which we know is a buildup of abnormal collagen). Cosmeceutical copper peptides promise to heal aging skin in a similar way: by promoting collagen, elastin, and GAG synthesis. It also boasts the added benefit of having potent antioxidant properties to quell free radicals.

The Facts: Copper peptides have indeed been shown to be wound-healing facilitators. It is true that the wound-healing process is similar physiologically to rejuvenating aging skin. Copper is also a coenzyme for collagen synthesis, in the same way that niacinamide is cofactor for the reaction that increases ceramide production in the skin. It also triggers an enzyme involved in cross-linking collagen and elastin. The ingredient has been found in vitro to induce production of the extracellular "packing foam" in the dermis—collagen, elastin, and GAGs. Copper also stimulates the enzyme super-oxide dismutase, a powerful antioxidant in the skin, and has anti-inflammatory properties.

Like all good things, many medications and topical ingredients included, too much can be dangerous. Because it fuels enzymes (the workers in the body's recycling program), the right amount can trigger production of new collagen and elastin, as well as the healthy removal of abnormal collagen (scar tissue). But excess copper in the system can trigger free-radical damage and increase MMP proliferation, ironically degrading the extracellular matrix and accelerating skin aging—the exact opposite effect of what it can do in the right quantity.

My Bottom Line: Because copper is vital to enzyme function in the body, it follows that it's also important to the synthesis of the extracellular matrix in the skin. I sound like a broken record, but although the notion of applying copper cutaneously to assist skin function is interesting in theory, it may be ineffectual in practice. Is there enough concentrated copper peptide in an over-the-counter product, and is it stable? Can it actually penetrate the skin to have an effect on the enzymatic workings of the body? Personally, I would rather eat foods containing copper (such as sesame, sunflower seeds, and cashews) to be sure the element is getting into my body to do its amazing job.

👎 I'm doubtful until much stronger scientific data proves the claims.

Beauty Pills:
Can Nutriceuticals Fight Skin Aging from the Inside Out?

Since cosmetic companies are always devising new ingredients and innovative ways to get them into the skin, it's inevitable that cosmetic nutritional supplements are the logical next step. Why not also ingest those antioxidants and fatty acids, doubling their power by using them internally and externally? Consumers seem to buy it. In 2005, Americans spent about $50 million on nutricosmetics, according to Kline & Company, a market research firm. In chapter 4, I advised that eating a healthy diet is a more efficient way to get the nutrients necessary to improve skin since the body metabolizes food better than it does pills. For many, it's easier and perhaps more satisfying to swallow some capsules rather than eat a plate of vegetables. You think and hope that the supplements you ingest carry the same magical power of a beauty product you apply. You might believe that a few doses of antioxidant pills or omega-3 fatty acids will have your skin looking hydrated and youthful in no time. I hate to burst that bubble, but—just as with cosmetics—it's difficult to know if these nutritional supplements really work since most research is done in-house and remains unpublished. And as with cosmeceuticals, the FDA does not vet supplements since they are classified as foods, not pharmaceuticals.

Physiologically speaking, only a minimal amount of the nutrients in a vitamin supplement ever reaches the skin. Excess vitamin C, for instance, is eliminated from the body before it ever reaches the periphery of the dermis or the epidermis. It sounds as though systemic ingredients have just as difficult a journey as their topical siblings. Though research has shown that ingesting green tea seems to reduce the incidence of skin cancer (at least in mice) and taking oral vitamins C and E for three months can reduce UV damage, there's not much science to support the taking of supplements to reduce wrinkles.

Pills aren't the only internal delivery system either. There are green tea mints, nutrient-packed waters, antioxidant elixirs, and tinctures. *The New York Times* reported in a 2006 story on nutricosmetics that a Japanese company makes "collagen marshmallows that claim to plump the skin and in France they sell gourmet anti-aging jam in flavors like tomato–green tea."

These herbs and botanicals may seem healthy and relatively harmless, but it's important to remember that they can be harmful or interact with medication that you are taking. It is possible to take too much of a certain nutrient or herb, and it could possibly become toxic in your body. When it comes to innovative (albeit natural) new chemicals, how can we be sure they aren't dangerous? For example, resveratrol is a promising antioxidant that has been proven to extend longevity in mice, but one study found that it might stimulate the proliferation of breast cancer cells.[15] Another showed that it did just the opposite, inhibiting estrogen and preventing breast cancer.[16] On some level, I think we're in danger of making our bodies (and our faces) a Petri dish of chemicals, many of which are untested. If your diet is poor, it's a good idea to talk to your doctor about using supplements to improve it, but you can't radically transform your skin by popping vitamins.

>>> q&a

Q: Can face creams that claim to work like Botox really do that?

A: No. If they did, I suppose we'd all be using them. Consider that the neurotoxin botulinum type A (Botox, PureTox, and other new formulations) is injected directly into a muscle to block its nerve receptors and temporarily paralyze it. A topical product has low odds of penetrating to the dermis and zero chance of reaching the muscle. So how can these creams and lotions possibly relax muscle contractions? Many of these Botox-lite products contain a synthetic hexapeptide called Argireline (acetyl hexapeptide-3), which theoretically works by inhibiting neurotransmitters that signal muscles to contract. Another ingredient is GABA, or gamma-aminobutyric acid, a neurotransmitter found in the body's nervous system. GABA analogs are used in anti-anxiety medication, and they act in a similar way to Argireline in cosmetic use—as a muscle relaxant. Since GABA can't penetrate the skin, cosmetic chemists add a plant extract to assist it. Even so, it's a tall order for any topical beauty product to inhibit nerve-to-muscle signals in the body. Can the long-term use of either of these ingredients accumulate deeply enough to soften expression lines? If they did, since these creams aren't able to target muscles selectively as Botox does, all the muscles in your face could be rendered expressionless. (Perhaps it's a good thing that penetration of topical cosmeceuticals is unlikely!) The latest ingredient to enter this line-smoothing race is manganese gluconate, a mineral found in the body. Topically applied, it is supposed to diminish wrinkles by preventing fibroblast cells from contracting. What? You know by now that the fibroblasts' job is to produce collagen. These cells do not create wrinkles; only repeated muscle contractions and a gradual depletion of the extracellular matrix can do that. With little scientific research to validate all these claims, I'd rather spend my money on the real thing. Botox injections provide almost immediate gratification and a controlled, positive outcome that is certain.

Q: I've heard about stem cell creams and products that repair DNA. Do they work? Are they safe?

A: The last question is valid, if indeed these products do work. After all, they claim to do such things as activate the synthesis of stem cells, reprogram them, or interfere with DNA replication in some way. If they did what they promise, they could definitely be dangerous and might even cause mutations that could lead to cancer. (The ingredients in these products would also be considered pharmaceuticals by law.) The research on both skin care technologies is relatively new, and as of now, I consider them unproven.

Stem cell creams don't contain stem cells. Like most cosmeceuticals, the science behind the ingredients relies on re-creating an element already in the body. One technology incorporates a synthetically engineered enzyme called telomerase, which prevents cell mutations and assists in DNA replication in the body. As a topical ingredient, it's supposed to activate the production of stem cells in the skin. (Back to Chapter 1: these are the pluripotential cells that have the ability to develop into any kind of cell when called upon to repair or maintain tissue.) Another stem cell cream utilizes a polypeptide to stimulate stem cells into differentiating. I have yet to see strong, objective scientific studies that prove that either of these ingredients is able to penetrate the skin and interact with stem cell synthesis.

DNA repair products aim to get into cells and fix DNA damage using bioengineered enzymes (some are derived from ocean plankton and encapsulated in a microsphere that allegedly penetrates the skin and releases the enzymatic ingredient). The same biotechnology company that manufactures this OTC cosmeceutical has developed Dimericine, a topical pharmaceutical that utilizes enzymes that mimic the body's own to repair DNA damage after UV exposure. While Dimericine is undergoing clinical trials for FDA approval as a drug to suppress the development of skin cancers, its cosmeceutical sister—which draws on natural ocean enzymes—is on the market as a remedy for photoaging. The idea behind this is based on true science. In the late 1990s, Barbara Gilchrest of Boston University School of Medicine and her team studied how applying tiny snippets of DNA to skin cells in vitro (and in rodent experiments) spurred cells to repair DNA damage from UV light faster. Perhaps cosmetic chemists latched onto that fascinating information and devised a way to manipulate it, or maybe they have discovered something truly amazing. The facts remain to be seen, but for now I would prefer to trust my own enzymes to repair my DNA and rely on my body's stem cells to know when and how to develop and specialize.

Q: Is it safe to use retinoic acid while I'm pregnant, or should I switch to an over-the-counter retinol product temporarily?

A: I would stay away from both. In fact, I recommend curtailing the use of most cosmeceuticals during pregnancy. Natural ingredients are essentially chemicals too. None of them has been scientifically tested with the kind of adequacy that would make me believe that they are 100 percent safe, and studies have not been conducted on the effects they may have on pregnant women. Retinoic acid is a drug and should not be taken during pregnancy because it could potentially be toxic to a fetus. (Note that isotretinoin, a systemic form of the vitamin A derivative, is completely forbidden for pregnant women and could cause birth defects.) The same goes for prescription hydroquinone, salicylic acid, and benzoyl peroxide. I tell my patients to stop chemical peels, Botox, fillers, everything during this time. (Lasers, however, are safe during pregnancy because they don't introduce a chemical into your body.) Glycolic and lactic acid products are considered nontoxic since they are derived from foods such as fruit and milk. Sunscreen appears to be safe, and since sun and hormonal changes trigger melasma, it's important to use it every day. Be on the safe side and ask your ob/gyn about anything that you think might be harmful.

>>> skin lie: Serums penetrate the skin better than creams or lotions do.

>>> skin truth: Marketing departments are always devising sensible reasons for us to buy something new and unnecessary. According to magazine articles and cosmetic advertisements, a serum should be layered underneath a moisturizer since it has a more concentrated composition of ingredients. Okay. But the fact is that a serum is not necessarily stronger than a lotion or cream delivery system. And since the label doesn't tell us the concentration of ingredients, we can't be sure if it is more potent. Some serums are oil-based, some are water-based, some might allow the ingredients to

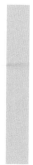

remain more stable, and some may be more compatible with the skin. Serums (like every other product on the shelves) are not created equal, but it's difficult to gauge any of this because cosmeceutical labels don't provide enough information. Perhaps an unstable ingredient (such as vitamin C) may remain stable in a serum formulation containing fewer inactive ingredients. If so, layering it underneath a sunscreen might make sense. In general, I think a serum is just another layer, another product to purchase, and more time you have to spend on your face.

>>> q&a

Q: I've heard that oxygen facials are good for the skin and make it look radiant. Are oxygen skin care products just as effective?

A: Of all the amazing things the skin can do, breathing is not one of them. Oxygen, as a topical ingredient, is completely ineffectual. Although I'm sure that an oxygen facial makes your skin glowing and radiant, the effect has nothing to do with oxygen. The machine used for this facial treatment has a hose-like attachment that discharges pressurized oxygen along with a hydrating hyaluronic acid serum. The moisturizing mist is what plumps the skin and makes it temporarily look and feel dewy. The use of oxygen cosmetically claims to have a wound-healing effect on the skin. This may stem from the fact that hyperbaric oxygen treatment has been proven to help heal wounds, but placing a patient in a hyperbaric chamber to increase the amount of oxygen in the lungs, which in turn delivers it through the blood to injured tissue, is not the same as having air and water sprayed onto your face. It is impossible to infuse skin cells with oxygen from the outside. It cannot purify or moisturize the skin, although too much oxygen has been known to generate toxic oxygen radicals that damage skin. For that matter, I have no idea how a cream or lotion could contain a stabilized form of oxygen, which is a gas. Carefully reading the explanations of cosmetic claims can be entertaining. They often make little logical sense. In this case, the science behind oxygen as a skin care ingredient is pretty easy to see through.

Q: Why are so many antiaging face creams so expensive? Are they better than the cheaper products at the drugstore?

A: Like most other aspects of beauty and fashion, price is subjective. Often it has more to do with marketing and pretty packaging than what's inside, even though advertising touts the ingredients as miracle workers. Manufacturers tell you that the price is high because the ingredients are exotic and precious (rare Japanese seaweed, shark cartilage, argan oil from Morocco, Arctic cranberries) or bioengineered synthetic copies of natural elements (amino acids harvested from human placenta, growth factors cultivated from the breast milk of cows or from fetal foreskin). There are some pretty bizarre ingredients (usually they are analogs, or man-made duplicates of the real thing) that push the price up, and the more outlandish the more expensive. Does that synthetic peptide replicating the venom of a Southeast Asian temple viper really work like Botox? If the synthetic snake venom doesn't grab us, perhaps we'll pay up for a night cream with an emollient that mimics the sap from cedar trees in far-off, drought-subjected continents. So one factor in the cost could definitely be research and development of these unusual items (and travel expenses too, I assume).

Sexy and scientific ingredients aside, prestige brands do offer intelligent (and patented) combinations of synergistic ingredients, or use high-tech methods of delivery (such as microsphere encapsulation and nanotechnology) that are proprietary and that may work well. It's also true that often you're really paying for a beautiful jar of something luxurious to display in the bathroom. If that motivates you to use the moisturizer every night and makes you feel wonderful when you put it on, it's worth the cash, in my opinion.

Keep in mind that drugstore products have some high-powered backup too. Remember that Procter & Gamble's beauty research team is over two thousand strong. L'Oréal, the drugstore mainstay that includes Maybelline, Garnier Nutritioniste, and La Roche-Posay, also owns the prestige brands Lancôme, Kiehl's, SkinCeuticals, and Shu Uemura. One certainly imagines that all these cosmetic giants pool their knowledge, information, laboratories, and ingredients. A 2007 *Consumer Reports* test found that luxury brands didn't work any better than drugstore products. In fact, the publication's top-rated product line is available at drugstores. Ultimately, a beauty purchase is all about personal preference. What a product looks or smells like makes all the difference. But when it comes to efficacy and ingredients, it doesn't have to cost a fortune.

Q: Are skin care lines created by famous dermatologists better than other brands?

A: Yes and no. First of all, just because they are developed and endorsed by doctors, that doesn't make them prescription strength by any means. As with makeup artist brands or professional hair stylist lines, dermatologists back up their products with their expertise and years of know-how. So their professional reputation is on the line. Consumers definitely respond to personal brand names. According to the market research company NPD Group, 28 percent of female skin care users eighteen and older said they prefer brands that have a physician's endorsement. Having a doctor's name either on the label or endorsing a product substantiates its validity as we tend to trust what doctors tell us. Some doctor brands may actually be better because they are believed in, developed and researched by the physician. Also, doctors get direct and immediate feedback from their patients. If they try a new product and have a bad reaction, it will be improved and perfected immediately. In a way, this a valuable human-controlled clinical test. It's a privilege to hear and see those real responses, which is something huge corporations lack. There are pros and cons to all different kinds of skin care products, and the one thing to remember is that most creams and lotions are essentially pretty similar: for the most part they are safe, but they are not the skin-transforming, life-changing fountains of youth that we'd love them to be.

10

The Big Breakthroughs:
Cosmetic Procedures That Deliver

The Choice Game: Botox, Fillers, Peels, and Lasers—
Which Wins You Younger Skin?

I t goes back to the feeling I had when I broke that paddle and used it to splint a camper's fractured leg when I was leading canoe trips after college. I get the same excitement when someone comes to my office and says, "I feel like I look older and tired, what can I do?" I know I have the skill and the tools to help them look and feel better. Even with the cosmetic aspect of my job, I am essentially a problem solver. In a medical case, such as skin cancer, the consequences are more critical—sometimes a matter of life and death. With cosmetic dermatology, the results enable a person to become more confident, powerful, and happy. Both situations are important, and I treat them (and all my patients) with the same therapeutic respect.

The ramifications of rejuvenation go deeper than the surface, in more ways than one. On a physical level, tools such as Botox, lasers, and dermal fillers can reliably and safely solve problems that have been bothering someone for years. Some procedures supply immediate gratification, such as zapping away brown spots or erasing lines, and some can provide long-term antiaging results by growing more collagen and invigorating the extracellular matrix. These procedures actually restore what is being lost with age, and they eliminate the bad stuff (wrinkles, sun damage, sagging) that comes fast and furious with each passing year, or sometimes it seems each month. The scientific breakthroughs in cosmetic dermatology are revolutionary, yet (in the hands of an artful physician) they produce subtle changes that allow a person to age naturally, and beautifully.

On the inside, the way you look definitely plays into how you feel, and I firmly believe that doing something proactive to improve both is not vanity but empowerment. Recently a woman in her sixties came to me for a cosmetic consultation. She'd been working hard and saving her money for many years to take a trip to Ireland. Instead, she decided to use that savings to make herself feel better in another way. She ended up getting fractional laser resurfacing, Botox, and dermal fillers—the dermatologic equivalent of a face lift without the surgery. When she was finished, she looked ten years younger and felt it too. She had no regrets and returned to work a more energized, positive person. Ironically, someone who had just seen her commented, "You must have had the best vacation, you look amazing!"

I notice that a lot of people look into cosmetic dermatology when they're switching jobs. They think an aesthetic improvement will make them feel stronger and more confident. And it will. In this youth-oriented society, an exhausted appearance doesn't give them an edge. (*The Wall Street Journal* recently reported that forty-something job seekers are taking dates and experience off their résumés to seem younger in the competitive market. Dermatologists do the same by taking years off of the face.) I see lots of women (and many men) who have to put their best face forward every day. To them, looking and feeling youthful are a matter of utility, not vanity. My patients who have procedures done to enhance their professional appearance are very concerned that no one be able to tell that they've had anything "done." They want zero downtime, no bruises, and gradual improvements that look natural. The goal: to appear magically refreshed and undetectably more youthful.

Cosmetic dermatology has become more mainstream for everyone, not just rich socialites, celebrities, and high-powered executives in New York or Los Angeles. People from all walks of life and every city in the country are more aware than ever of the noninvasive possibilities available for those who want them. The number of nonsurgical cosmetic procedures performed annually in the United States went from 1.1 million in 1997 to 9.6 million in 2007, according to the American Society of Plastic Surgeons, and that year Americans spent $4.7 billion on them.

All this is certainly not to say that everyone needs to have work done and filler injected at a certain age. When is it something to consider? Maybe never. There's no reason to be self-critical. If it hasn't occurred to you, you don't need it. I would not suggest that if you have some wrinkles you necessarily need Botox. But if you are focused on them, or on lax skin or brown spots, there are solutions. If you're spending serious money on skin care products that may take forever to render results, and if you look in the mirror and are dissatisfied with what you see, there are many options available that can help.

I'm aware that having substances injected into your face or having lasers or acids used on it seem pretty far from "simple skin beauty." But in all honesty, going to a dermatologist for one treatment or a short series of them can save you money, time, and loads of frustration in the long run. I hear so many patients complain that their brown spots haven't faded, even after months of diligent use of hydroquinone. Lasers can fix them. Or they wonder why monthly enzyme peels by a facialist aren't doing anything to brighten their skin or get rid of sun damage. That's when a stronger chemical peel or fractional laser resurfacing can literally transform their complexion.

Without a doubt, all of the procedures I discuss in this chapter are relatively expensive. But if you calculate all the products you've purchased, the facials you've had, and the time you've spent on your skin, it probably exceeds the amount of money and time it takes to have one or two laser treatments and be done with it. Having sun spots taken off with a laser, a face full of sun damage treated with peels or laser treatments, or wrinkles relaxed with Botox is simple, dependable, and efficient. I consider the short- and long-term benefits to be a great investment.

For most of us, beauty is all about upkeep. It's plain old hard work, and it gets harder as we get older. In *Bridget Jones's Diary,* Helen Fielding's everywoman heroine writes, "Being a woman is worse than being a farmer—there is so much harvesting and crop spraying to be done: legs to be waxed, underarms shaved, eyebrows plucked, feet pumiced, skin exfoliated and moisturized, spots cleansed, roots dyed, eyelashes tinted, nails filed, cellulite massaged. The whole performance is so highly tuned you only need to neglect it for a few days for the whole thing to go to seed. Is it any wonder girls have no confidence?"

As we get older, working the land is even more essential to keep the crops from failing—or falling, if the face and skin are the harvest we're trying to save. Topical products (especially sunscreen) are essential to maintaining your skin's integrity and saving it from brown spots, fine lines, and premature aging and averting the need for more serious dermatologic attention, at least for a while. Eventually, however, the aging process sneaks up and begins to show (even vigilant use of sunscreen can't stop gravity and the biological clock from altering your skin and facial structure). At this point topical solutions (which work primarily on the surface levels of your skin) aren't going to provide noticeable results fast enough. Not even retinoic acid is going to plump and firm your skin in a matter of days or even weeks. This is where dermatologic intervention can accomplish things that no product can: by vaporizing spots, erasing lines, resurfacing the skin, and literally building collagen.

Cosmetic dermatologists have supreme confidence in the safety, efficacy, and power of these techniques. If we did not believe they work, we wouldn't recommend them. A cosmetic practice demands an extraordinary monetary investment on the part of a physician. Just one laser can cost approximately $200,000. The protective eyewear for each laser costs upward of $1,000, since the glasses are different for each machine and everyone who is in the room during a procedure must wear them. Fillers and Botox also involve huge initial expenses for the doctor. Plus we use special, tiny needles that make injections less painful, sterile syringes, and all the best medical materials. The overhead adds up quickly! Just to get started injecting, a dermatologist needs to invest about $10,000. So if one device or injectable isn't effective or safe, we certainly won't purchase it or use it on our patients. We spend a lot of effort and money to perfect the experience for patients and make them more comfortable.

Once upon a time (less than ten years ago), restoring a moderately sagging neck or jowls meant having a neck lift. Crow's feet, sunken eyes, and the downward pull of gravity on the face could only be altered with surgery too. There were no other options. Now brilliant therapies combining Botox, filler, and laser treatments can dramatically improve these problems with no general anesthesia, no scalpel, and much less recovery time. These options are liberating for people who don't want to go under the knife. The advances in cosmetic procedures can allow a dermatologist to sculpt the face, enhancing cheekbones with dermal filler or injecting filler into the chin to balance the overall shape of the face. This can replace the need for surgical implants. My patients are relieved to be able to stave off a surgical overhaul or avoid it completely. It's not too surprising that of the 11.5 million cosmetic procedures performed in 2006, more than four in five were noninvasive treatments, according to the Aesthetic Plastic Surgery Society. In 2006, the number of face-lifts dropped by 5 percent, while the number of minimally invasive procedures increased by 53 percent to 8.4 million, according to the American Society of Plastic Surgeons.

Noninvasive cosmetic procedures improve the structure of the face and the quality of the skin through subtle alterations. A millimeter change here or there will make a person appear younger but still look natural. Even so, such modifications (with filler or Botox) won't be enough in some cases. When skin is extremely slack and sagging (on the upper eyelids or at the neck), even the most extreme nonsurgical treatments won't be able to repair it to the patient's satisfaction. This is when surgery is the best answer, and I encourage my patients to have it done. I've worked with people who would have been better off getting a face-lift but flat-out refused to have one. They wanted fillers and Botox to transform them. Ultimately, even though their procedures were successful, they were disappointed because they wanted more dramatic results.

By the same token, a face-lift won't do anything for dull, sun-damaged skin or brown spots. For this reason, the plastic surgery and dermatology fields overlap. Plastic surgeons often augment and fine-tune surgical work with dermatologic procedures. A brow lift, for example, is enhanced when Botox erases the crow's feet (which surgery can't soften), and it can prolong the surgical results since Botox suppresses the movements that help cause wrinkles in the first place. Often, while a patient is under general anesthesia for a face-lift, the surgeon does a chemical peel too. As procedures become less invasive, procedural dermatologists (this dermatologic field includes face-lifts, vascular procedures, liposuction, etc.) are pioneering more and more surgical techniques. Did you know that dermatologists developed liposuction? Some leading plastic surgeons predict the future merging of the two fields. Surgical and noninvasive techniques work hand in hand to enhance each other's effectiveness. And at home, the use of topical products (especially sunscreen and moisturizer) will protect and preserve the positive effects of any cosmetic procedure. Ah, we can't get away from maintenance and upkeep altogether.

Finding a Cosmetic Dermatologist

Start your search with your own dermatologist's recommendation (sometimes a primary care physician can lead you in the right direction too). Or begin by checking the listings of dermatologists who specialize in cosmetic work on the American Academy of Dermatology Web site (www.aad.org) or the American Society for Dermatologic Surgery Web site (www.asds.net). I don't think media are necessarily the best way to find a doctor (and celebrity dermatologists can have very long waiting lists to see new patients). You're better off with someone who has an academic affiliation, who's been in practice for several years, and who is fellowship-trained in cosmetic dermatology.

Word of mouth is great but a little tricky. Finding a terrific cosmetic dermatologist is not as politically correct as inquiring about someone's hairstylist. You can't exactly ask, "Who does your Botox?" You can start the conversation with a few trusted friends, and you might be surprised at their answers. Someone you thought was genetically blessed (or younger than you thought) may refer you to a terrific cosmetic dermatologist, since her youthful-looking skin is due partially to that doctor's expertise.

The Consultation

Once you've located one or two candidates, schedule a consultation. You won't insult one physician by meeting with another before you make a decision. Speaking with more than one doctor is important and accepted protocol. (Consultations can be expensive. You might ask the doctor if you can apply the consultation fee toward your first treatment if you schedule it within two weeks.) There's no reason to downplay the choice of who will best be able to artfully and safely inject fillers or Botox into your face or help you decide between a chemical peel and laser resurfacing. You have to feel confident about a doctor's experience and comfortable with him or her as a person. If a doctor doesn't give you more than a few minutes of time, doesn't thoroughly explain procedures or their side effects, treats you with condescension, or won't answer all of your questions thoughtfully, that's a sign to move on to another doctor. Any cosmetic procedure is significant and serious enough to warrant a doctor's listening to your concerns and addressing them. Also examine the office: Is the space clean? Is the staff professional and well organized? Remember, when it comes to cosmetic rejuvenation, it's rarely a one-shot deal (pardon the pun). Botox, fillers, laser treatments, and peels must all be repeated eventually—whether in a series of sessions or because the treatment wears off (as Botox does). It's important to trust your dermatologist, to like the office atmosphere and the support staff, and to feel safe there. The experience should be a positive one.

Besides exemplary medical experience, another important qualification for a cosmetic dermatologist is aesthetic skill. Working with injectables is an art. I feel almost like a sculptor when I'm working on someone's face. When I look at a patient, I can visualize what the perfect amount of filler would be and where it should be injected. When I perform the procedure, there's an almost imperceptible shift in the tissue when I've hit the sweet spot, and that's when I stop. This knowledge comes from years of experience. Even doing lasers and peels is something of an art form. It's not just going over the face with a light or applying acid to it. With a laser, I can stack the pulses or go over an area several times to get the result I want. With peels, I may do three passes on a particular section or use two different types of acids to achieve the most even effects. A talented cosmetic dermatologist knows the desired end result and how to achieve it, and uses his or her years of know-how and good judgment to choose the best procedures for each patient's individual needs.

During a consultation, you can ask to see before-and-after photos of a doctor's patients' results, but many dermatologists don't have such a portfolio. Some patients want total confidentiality, so showing their photos is inappropriate. Images can be touched up, and only the very best cases are chosen to show. Albums may be spectacular, but you can't always be sure they show the doctor's personal work. Simply talking to the doctor during a consultation may give you a better sense of his or her proficiency. Ask how many times a week he or she performs the procedure you want to have done. If he or she administers a lot of Botox injections on a regular basis, for instance, there's a greater chance that he or she is experienced in and especially expert at that technique.

Ask questions. Don't be afraid of offending a doctor with intelligent queries—as long as it doesn't become a long-winded interrogation. Usually a consultation lasts fifteen to twenty minutes. Ask for literature; most offices have prepared handouts that explain the procedures. Do your research beforehand—or read this chapter—to educate yourself about the procedures you are interested in. (Beware, though, of doing excessive Internet research; there's a lot of misinformation out there.) If you're thinking about getting laser treatments, ask how many different kinds of lasers the doctor has in the office. Many have only one or two—and now that you're aware of the cost, it's easy to understand why. If a laser that targets pigment will be more effective for your skin concerns than an intense pulsed light device, the doctor should be forthright about it. (But it's up to you to ask specific questions.) Generally, doctors won't recommend a procedure they don't think will be effective. They want to feel that they've done the best job they can for you.

Don't Forget to Ask

Will the doctor be doing the procedure?

This seems obvious, but many busy dermatologists don't perform every procedure themselves. Find out if they have a registered nurse, a nurse practitioner, or a physician extender do them. Don't be intimidated to insist that the doctor administer your treatment if it's associated with any risks. (Microdermabrasion is so safe that it doesn't have to be performed by the doctor.)

What side effects or complications may occur, and how would the doctor manage them? What are the risks?

If the doctor says he or she has never had a side effect, he or she is not telling the truth or hasn't done many procedures. With almost every procedure there is a little bruising and some swelling, redness, and pain. The risks may also involve scarring (such as hyper- or hypopigmentation) or infection.

What can I expect during the procedure? What should I do before and afterward?

I'll go over that later in this chapter, but the doctor should walk you through it.

And Ask Yourself

The consultation is your chance to ask questions and start a frank discussion with your dermatologist about what you'd like to change right away and where you see yourself in the future. So ask *yourself* the following questions; then you will communicate better with the physician.

What are my goals?

The first thing a patient needs to know is what he or she wants to look like. During a consultation, I hand the patient a big mirror and ask "What can I do for you? When you look in the mirror, what would you most like to change?" Most people throw the question back at me and reply, "But what do you think I need to do?" It's difficult to see yourself objectively, and your self-perception is deeply rooted in your personality and your own life, so I understand how difficult that question can be. Bring a photograph of yourself (a flattering shot from five or ten years ago that you love). This is a great tool for conveying your goals to the doctor.

What is my budget?

Figure out the amount you've allotted to spend beforehand, and do your homework on the current costs of various procedures so you're prepared. (Remember that many, such as peels and laser treatments, require a series of appointments.) Once you decide on a potential course of action, ask your doctor if it's realistic to accomplish it on your budget. Perhaps it's due to all the makeover shows on television or the breezy magazine articles about cosmetic procedures, but many patients mistakenly believe that cosmetic dermatology is like waving a magic wand over the face and making it look younger for $300 or less with no pain and no downtime. None of these things is true. It is a process, it will be relatively painful, there will be some recovery time involved (even if it's minimal), and will not be cheap.

What are my expectations?

It's important to understand and appreciate the limitations of what these procedures can do. They cannot remake you into a new person. That's why I ask people to bring a picture of themselves, not some movie star they wish they looked like. (Funnily enough, most of my patients say they don't want lips like Angelina Jolie, even though she's drop-dead gorgeous. For the most part, people don't really want to look that different.) If total transformation is what you want, I'm not going to be able to achieve that goal, nor do I want to. My goal is to capture your own individual beauty and enhance it in subtle ways, to make you look fresher and more youthful, not to change your face. Most people are focused on one or two features that they dislike (and probably always have). But there are some women (and men) who are unhappy and self-critical about the way they look in general. They overemphasize every detail of their face and want to perfect each perceived flaw—a psychological condition called body dysmorphic disorder. Sometimes patients come to see me during a traumatic time in their lives, for example, after the loss of a loved one or during a divorce, and I can tell that they want to change who they are, not just rejuvenate their skin. This leads to impulsive decisions, and I advise them to put off having a procedure done for now. I also recommend that they visit one of my psychologist colleagues, who can help them handle the stress in their lives.

What are my fears?

Duck lips and a frozen face. These are the biggest fears I hear about, and I completely understand them! Most people are terrified that they're going to end up looking like a plastic mask (we've all seen those cosmetic-procedures-gone-overboard photos in the tabloids). This is why it's so important to find the right physician and to have an open dialogue with him or her. As a cosmetic dermatologist, I think that part of my balancing act is preventing people from going too far. My job is to be an honest gatekeeper, the voice of reason advising patients when to back off and do less in order to look natural. I frequently dissuade patients from having too much done, erasing every line and all expression. I used to show some of them a picture of my newborn son to demonstrate that even babies have nasolabial folds, the creases that run from each side of the nose down to the corners of the mouth. To remove every facial feature looks alien.

If you're afraid of the pain of a procedure or what the outcome might be, this is when you should tell us. When I'm comfortable with patients' expectations, if they understand the side effects, what it will feel like, and what the results will be, I know I can reassure them and do a better job.

Where *Not* to Go for Dermatologic Procedures

Procedures are becoming so mainstream that more and more "medical spas" (or "medspas") are popping up all over the country. The International Medical Spa Association estimates that there are up to 2,500 medspas nationwide. "Laser centers" and medspas are set up in minimalls right next to banks and Starbucks. (Norwegian Cruise Lines even announced that it is offering Botox and injectable fillers in its ships' medspas.) It does seem convenient (grab a coffee and your dry cleaning and get a laser treatment), but these derm franchises and the Botox parties they are throwing are a dangerous, albeit booming, business. In most medspas, the staff can legally use filler, do Botox, and perform laser treatments, all without any proper medical training. A medical aesthetician goes through a training course but is not a nurse or a doctor. Most medspas have aestheticians or nurses administer Botox and filler injections, chemical peels, and laser treatments. These are serious medical procedures with very real risks—a far cry from getting a haircut or a facial at a spa. Often an MD is not even on the premises to supervise or intercede if an emergency or a complication occurs. I've had to treat people who are left with scars from laser treatments done by a spa technician.

Non-MDs aren't as aware of important details that can cause ill effects. They probably won't ask if a client uses retinoids, which can cause a reaction with a peel or laser. They may not ask if the client is tan, in which case lasers can trigger hyperpigmentation. When I had fractionated laser surfacing done by a doctor, a small area on my nose (the location of my scar from skin cancer surgery) turned white. An aesthetician, or even a trained nurse, may not notice that or know how to respond, and this could lead to worse scarring. A filler may be incorrectly injected into a major artery and block it, causing skin ulceration and scars. I know prestigious doctors to whom this happened, but they know how to deal with that kind of emergency immediately. My medical colleagues, respected professionals who have been doing cosmetic procedures for years, are still learning and perfecting new ways to inject Botox. This is a medical technique *and* an art form. Translate that kind of expertise to someone in a lab coat at a medspa who has taken a Botox and dermal filler training course. Whom do you feel safer receiving a cosmetic procedure from? Not to mention that I've recognized early skin cancers in patients who've come in to have a brown spot lasered off when it's actually a melanoma. An aesthetician will likely overlook an indication of a serious problem like that.

Government regulation of how much medical training is required to perform cosmetic procedures differs from state to state. A new medical spas bill sponsored by the American Society for Dermatologic Surgery will hopefully be passed soon in California. It prohibits nonphysicians from performing any procedures without a physician on site unless the treatment is performed in a physician-owned office. This legislation will set an important precedent for other states to follow. Florida has already enacted a similar law that states that only dermatologists and plastic surgeons can supervise a medical spa, not ER physicians, orthopedic surgeons, etc. The American Society for Dermatologic Surgery has seen an increase in the number of patients treated for complications from cosmetic procedures performed by nonphysicians, which is why this group is so adamant about passing stricter regulations to protect the consumers' safety.

There have also been instances of black-market Botox and fillers imported from unreliable sources and physicians (and aestheticians) who pay house calls to inject Botox in a mobile spa setting. I've seen deep fungal infections and nodules that arose because injections were done in a nonsterile setting. This is major-league medical stuff and should not be taken lightly. It pays to protect your skin and your health by having procedures such as Botox, filler, laser (including IPL light treatments and laser hair removal), even moderate chemical peels (with any acid over 10% concentration) administered in a medical environment by a physician.

>>> q&a

Q: What does it mean when Botox, a filler, or a cosmetic treatment is used "off label"? Is this unsafe or illegal?

A: Using drugs or medical devices off label is common and considered legal and safe when a medical doctor does it. Botox is classified as a drug and has gone through all the trials that a pharmaceutical requires. FDA approval is based on scientific studies with exact hypotheses and conclusions. These trials must define the parameters and details regarding the safety of using a product in a very specific way. Botox is expressly approved "on label" for reducing frown lines between the eyebrows. But dermatologists use it all the time elsewhere on the face—on crow's feet, under the eyes, all over the forehead, even on the neck. It's also used under the arms and on the palms of the hands to decrease sweating (and it works!). These are all "off-label" uses, meaning it's used for an indication that's not specifically FDA-approved. The hyaluronic acid filler Restylane is approved as a medical device for use on the nasolabial folds of people with Types 3 to 6 skin color, for example. But doctors legitimately use it on other areas of the face or body off label. The FDA states that physicians can legally use a drug or medical device (including lasers and fillers) using "their best knowledge and judgment, and in the best interests of the patient."

FDA approval of devices such as lasers and dermal fillers is based on safety alone. Oddly enough, fillers are considered to be "medical devices" (just like laser machines) by the FDA, which is why companies are able to push through approval at a relatively rapid pace. This is a little scary on one hand but positive on another. The rules for drug approval are so rigid that it would be a prohibitively expensive and protracted process to go through trials of each new laser or filler, and there would probably not be as many options available on the market. Since a lot of fillers are tested in other countries before they are used in the United States, I think this system is good, albeit imperfect. (Europe and South America have an even more relaxed approval system than ours, so the number of cosmetic options in other continents is much greater.) Side effects and risks have already been reported in the European medical literature before we ever use a product here, so what makes it to the United States will be the safest ones. Of course, the physician's injection technique is equally essential for patient safety.

Aging and Facial Structure

It's not just fine lines and brown spots that indicate aging but the overall shape and balance of the face. Loss of elasticity and volume, decreased collagen, elastin, and even bone, and gravity all act to alter the symmetry of the face over time. The dissolving extracellular matrix is similar to a once-fluffy down pillow that eventually flattens and loses its shape. The ballast that cushions and supports your head is no longer as firm. Though peels and lasers make fast-acting changes to the surface of the skin, other procedures (such as laser resurfacing and especially injectables) work deeper to rebuild the extracellular matrix by initiating a wound-healing response that triggers the production of more collagen and elastin to fix the injury.

A cosmetic dermatologist evaluates a patient's face as a whole and also mentally assesses it in thirds, and will make recommendations using that template. Imagine a youthful face as an inverted triangle: the widest part goes from your forehead to your eyes, the middle third consists of the eyes to the mouth, and the lowest part is the mouth and chin area. All these thirds overlap with each other. As we age, the pyramid shape gradually turns upside down into more of a squared-off trapezoid. The lower third gets heavier as gravity pulls it downward, and what was once the widest third (the upper face) starts to sink and become thinner.

In medical terminology, we discuss cosmetic rejuvenation (especially when referring to injectables) in terms of these thirds of the face. For instance, we want to strengthen the weakening upper third and then balance out the overall structure. The fillers I use in the top third of the face are different from the fillers I inject in the middle (where there's more fat and denser tissue). If I do Botox in the upper third, it will elongate it a little bit, and that will change the dimensions, so I may want to do a touch of filler at the chin to add a millimeter of length to balance that out. As when designing your home, one change can lead to several others until the whole picture is balanced.

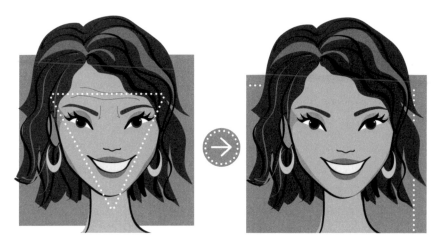

Younger face is triangular

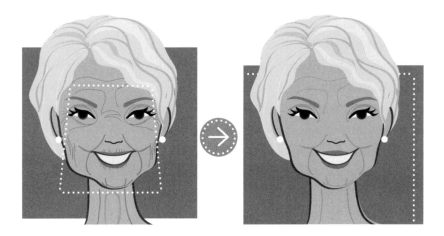

Mature face is trapezoidal

The shape of the face naturally changes with aging (or maturity).
Fillers can rejuvenate the shape and look of the face almost instantaneously.

The Choice Game

Every dermatologist has his or her own techniques and expert opinions about which procedure, or combination of therapies, will be most effective to achieve your goals within your budget. What will be the longest-lasting option or the safest for the patient's skin? Which requires the least downtime? Is this a more superficial problem of skin texture or a deeper one with a loss of volume in the dermis? With a wide array of tools at my disposal, I can address each issue more creatively. For instance, if someone has fine lines around the eyes and mouth and also has some sun damage, I'm going to choose between chemical peels and fractionated laser. If the patient were on a tight budget, peels would be the best way to go. If he or she is concerned about antiaging and sagging of the skin, I know that laser resurfacing will provide longer-lasting results since it builds collagen more effectively and will prevent more laxity in the future. This is part of the dialogue you should have with your physician, and it's obviously important for both parties to communicate clearly with each other.

Consider what follows to be a day in the life of my cosmetic practice. These are some of the choices I would make regarding a patient's treatment after I look at his or her facial structure and skin, and listen to what his or her particular problems or restrictions might be.

The Issue: Younger (twenty- or thirty-something) skin that's dull and a little sun-damaged.
My Choice: Microdermabrasion. This is the most superficial procedure I do in my office, so it won't provide much in the way of long-lasting benefits, but it smoothes and brightens the skin beautifully with absolutely no downtime. This is the procedure to have done before a big event (even right before your wedding).

The Issue: Fine lines around the mouth and eyes, dull skin, and a lot of sun damage.

My Choice: A series of moderate chemical peels. This is less expensive than having a fractionated laser treatment, but a deep enough peel can decrease wrinkles and definitely take care of hyperpigmentation. (Remember, I use 30% TCA peels to remove actinic keratoses, possible skin precancers.)

The Issue: Lots of fine lines and crow's feet, and the patient cannot take time off work to recover.
My Choice: Botox. The patient will see lines disappear (yes, they really do) in a matter of days and with zero downtime (a little bruising is the most common side effect).

The Issue: Aging skin with mild to moderate laxity and quite a bit of sun damage.
My Choice: Fractionated laser resurfacing works deep in the dermis to stimulate collagen and elastin production, but it's also a form of extreme exfoliation that restores the surface of the skin.

The Issue: A complexion with some sun damage, lots of freckles, and redness.
My Choice: Intense pulsed light (IPL) treatments are a great alternative for someone who doesn't need too much in the way of antiaging (perhaps a patient in his or her late thirties with overall firm, healthy skin). IPL is incredibly successful at treating rosacea, freckles, and especially poikiloderma—a mélange of white, brown, and red sun spots.

The Issue: A few brown spots here and there on the face (or anywhere).
My Choice: Pigment-specific lasers such as the Q-switched Nd: YAG can target spots precisely and literally vaporize them. Most of the time, one procedure does the trick. (A face full of sun spots is another story and might be better served with a chemical peel or laser resurfacing.)

The Issue: Dark, hollow eyes and an overall tired, Droopy Dog visage.
My Choice: Injectable fillers used in strategic areas—under the eyes and

in the nasolabial folds, the marionette lines—can make a gravity-defying change in volume that literally makes a face look ten years younger immediately.

Preparing for a Procedure

Except for microdermabrasion, consider all of these cosmetic treatments to be medical procedures, complete with pre-op and post-op instructions. The list below is the advice I pass along to my patients, and I urge them to follow these simple instructions. The procedure and recovery will go more smoothly, with less complication and risks and probably less pain too (now I have your attention).

What to Do and What to Avoid before You Have a Procedure

WITH EVERY TYPE OF TREATMENT

Stop using chemicals on your skin three days before. That means retinoids, acids, scrubs, benzoyl peroxide, and active ingredients in cosmeceuticals. The skin can react differently since it's already more sensitive or slightly irritated by these topical ingredients. This can create complications during the procedure or cause the doctor not to get the desired end result. Use the barest minimum for three days before and at least three days after, depending on the treatment you've had. (It's not a bad idea to also try sun protection with mineral sunblock such as zinc oxide or titanium dioxide, rather than chemical sunscreen ingredients.)

Take your makeup off before the procedure. This is most important with laser treatments, since the light source targets pigment and can interact with cosmetics on your skin. It's also smart to take it off before injections because makeup can be unsanitary.

If you are prone to herpes, fever blisters, or any kind of infection on your face (even acne), pretreat and posttreat it with the proper medication before and after your procedure. Any treatment can cause stress to the skin that may cause a flare-up of a skin condition. Most spas will not be able to manage these conditions that could cause terrible scars. This is a critical difference between doing procedures in a doctor's office and at a spa.

WITH INJECTABLES, BOTOX, AND LASERS

Discontinue all medically unnecessary blood-thinning medications and supplements one week before hand. (This includes aspirin, ibuprofen, St. John's wort, vitamin E, and omega-3 supplements.) This will help decrease bruising and bleeding. You can go back to using them three hours after the treatment. You can continue all prescription medications, including aspirin and warfarin, before these procedures; just know that you may have more bruising.

WITH LASERS

Don't be tan, and stop using self-tanner two weeks prior to treatment. Because lasers zone in on it, dark pigment in the skin can affect the outcome of the procedure and perhaps cause side effects such as postinflammatory hyperpigmentation. Consider that specialized pigment lasers are made to blow up melanosomes and will overreact to color in the skin, increasing your risk of side effects.

>>> 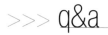 q&a

Q: Are all procedures painful, and why? Do any require a general anesthetic?

A: Except for microdermabrasion, they all hurt. Why? If a cosmetic procedure is supposed to induce collagen production and build the extracellular matrix, the skin will have to incur some kind of injury to the dermis, and that will necessitate some pain. Although this seems contradictory, lasers, light devices, peels, and even injectables all have to get down to the dermis and injure it to effect some kind of wound healing response that will make it stronger. For example, radiofrequency devices (such as Thermage) firm the skin by using heat to contract the tissue deep in the fat layer of the skin; that's got to hurt. But I've found (in myself and in my patients) that nothing motivates you to push through the pain more than a positive result—and that will happen once the pain is over with. Retrospective amnesia will no doubt set in later, and you will forget how much a procedure hurts in order to have it done again and get those results again. It's a little like having children; we'd never have more than one if not for retrospective amnesia about labor and delivery, and the joy we feel with the finished product.

As for the pain itself, this is a new era of pain management for cosmetic surgery, and there are now wonderful technologies and anesthetics to make a patient more comfortable. Because I happen to be a huge wimp, I put great emphasis on topical anesthetics before a procedure, and I also know that if a patient is comfortable the procedure will be more successful. Before a fractionated laser treatment, for example, a lidocaine paste is applied over the skin and it stays on for one hour to dull nerve receptors. (The procedure itself can take as little as ten minutes). High-tech lidocaine pastes can be used to numb the skin before all laser, peels, and injectable procedures. (Topical lidocaine will make the face red, but it's a welcome trade-off to pain.) Lidocaine injections (like a dental block, similar to the anesthetic shots you get at the dentist) are immensely helpful before injecting filler in the nasolabial folds, or marionette lines. In fact, lidocaine is even emulsified into some fillers, and some cosmetic dermatologists have the equipment (a special adaptor that attaches to a prefilled syringe) to mix lidocaine into filler themselves. These anesthesia-laced fillers really help minimize pain.

Every laser has some type of cooling mechanism attached that helps to alleviate the burning, stinging sensation involved in the process. It also keeps the epidermis from absorbing all the heat of the light source, so the laser doesn't dissipate all its energy in the top part of the skin before it can get to its deeper target. Fractionated laser machines have a Zimmer cooler, a separate hose-like attachment that sprays super-cold air over the skin as it's being lasered, numbing it at the same time. IPL uses contact cooling, a cold glass tip on the part of the device that touches the skin. A cold coupling gel (similar to the goo that's used on an ultrasound machine) is also applied to the glass tip to keep the light energy focused on a specific area, rather than spreading that sharp feeling over a larger area of skin.

Everyone has a different pain threshold. If you know yours is pretty low, tell your doctor beforehand that you need to be numbed with lidocaine. In my office, we apply numbing cream to anyone who wants it, even if the procedure isn't terribly painful. If you anticipate high anxiety or know you can't hack the pain, take a couple extra-strength Tylenol (not aspirin or ibuprofen) thirty minutes before the procedure, or bring a tranquilizer such as Valium with you and let your doctor know you want to take it beforehand. Ice packs are also a wonderful trick.

The Cosmetic Procedures

Welcome to the really exciting part of this book! (Those of you who skipped chapter 1—go back and read it now!) Each one of these procedure profiles describes the pain factor, recovery time, side effects, and length of time the results last. Note that all of these aspects are extremely variable. I have many patients who can sit through fractional laser resurfacing set at the highest energy level without flinching, while others (like me) can barely make it through at the lowest level for less than ten minutes. Everyone's pain threshold is different, and everyone's results or side effects will be too. Some patients don't have to get filler redone for well over one year (even though it's supposed to wear off in nine months), whereas some need a refill of a long-lasting injectable after only three months.

PAIN KEY

☺	NO PAIN
☹	NOT SO BAD
☹	OUCH
☹ ☹	IT HURTS
☹ ☹ ☹	IT'S TOTALLY PAINFUL
☹ ☹ ☹ ☹	THIS REALLY HURTS! HELP!

Microdermabrasion

What does it do? Microdermabrasion exfoliates the surface of the skin and smoothes the texture. It decreases the appearance of fine lines slightly since it lifts off dead skin, which lends a crumpled appearance to the surface layer. It's also an effective way to treat milia because it exfoliates all those tiny rough cysts. Microdermabrasion is also a terrific way to augment a peel, by exfoliating the peeling dead skin one week afterward.

How does it work? In the old days microdermabrasion employed crystals to sandblast the face, but that method has been replaced by an instrument with a rough, rounded tip that moves over the skin to polish it mechanically. It comes with various attachments that provide gentle to very aggressive exfoliation. (I've used the coarse tip to do dermabrasion scar revisions.) The device also incorporates pneumatic suction, so it vacuums up the debris as it sloughs it off. The gentle suction may even trigger some small amount of collagen production.

Who should try it? This is less a treatment for antiaging and brown spots and more for immediate gratification. It's a great way to get a radiant complexion with zero downtime. And for people with milia, I recommend regular microdermabrasion to keep them at bay. It's safe for dark skin too.

Who should not? Very inflamed acne or rosacea can be irritated by microdermabrasion. Anyone with extremely sensitive skin or active fever blisters or infections should not have the procedure done.

How long does it take? Fifteen to thirty minutes.

How does it feel? It's a massaging sensation—a gentle scraping along with simultaneous suction.

Pain factor: ☺

Side effects and recovery: People with sensitive skin may be a little pink for a few hours. Exfoliation like this tends to dry out the surface of the skin, so in my office we apply a rich moisturizing mask afterward, to rehydrate it. Follow up with your moisturizer at home if your face feels parched.

Social downtime: None.

When do you see results? Immediately. And your skin feels like silk!

How long does it last? Skin keeps renewing itself, so within approximately twenty-eight days the surface will begin to toughen up again. Exfoliating twice a week with either a chemical AHA or a mechanical scrub can preserve the skin-smoothing effects.

Postprocedure pearls: You must apply sunscreen before leaving the doctor's office, since freshly exfoliated skin is even more sensitive to the sun. Avoid using scrubs, acids, or retinoids on your face for two or three days for the same reason.

Follow-up sessions: Repeat treatments are not necessary, but they are desirable. Microdermabrasion provides a temporary effect, like having your hair highlighted. Every six weeks or so, you're going to wish you had another one. Some people get one every month.

Chemical Peels

What does it do? Most chemical peels work on a superficial level to exfoliate (by burning off) the top layers of skin. Peels can go down to the papillary dermis, which is the top part of the dermis. By doing so, a peel removes surface pigmentation (such as brown spots and melasma), smoothes the texture, decreases acne, and even helps firm the skin and reduces the appearance of fine lines. A strong peel, for example a 40% TCA peel, can go deeper into the dermis and cause enough inflammation to set up a wound healing response that can stimulate collagen formation.

How does it work? There are many types of peels—glycolic acid, retinoic acid, trichloracetic acid—and each has a different interaction with skin proteins and have varying specializations. TCA works on melanocytes; retinoic acid zones in on the sebaceous glands; lactic acid blows up keratinocytes and is an effective exfoliating agent; glycolic also exfoliates but has less risk of causing hyperpigmentation. Your dermatologist will choose the appropriate kind, and the concentration that will be safest and most effective for your particular skin type and conditions.

A higher concentration of acid will go deeper into the skin, disintegrating cells as it moves through. A lot of dermatologists do combination peels, combining two different acids at milder concentrations, rather than doing one super-intense peel, which can cause side effects or complications. For example, I may do three minutes of a 20% glycolic acid, wash it off, then do a 20% TCA. This is ultimately friendlier to sensitive skin types than working with one hard-core, highly concentrated peel—and easier for the patient to handle pain-wise.

Who should try it? TCA is "melanotoxic," destroying melanosomes that make pigment, so this kind of peel is ideal for treating melasma or superficial discoloration. A moderate chemical peel (20% to 30% TCA or 40% to 70% glycolic acid) is a less expensive way to improve your complexion with almost immediate gratification. It's the poor man's (or woman's, as the case may be) laser. Chemical peels are an effective way to tackle fine lines, dull skin, and sun damage with lots of brown spots. But only a robust (at least 30% TCA) peel will make significant changes to extremely sun-damaged skin with a loss of elasticity.

Who should not? Darker skin and Asian complexions (Fitzpatrick Types 3 to 6) are prone to ill effects—primarily postinflammatory hypo- or hyperpigmentation or PIH—from stronger peels, especially melanotoxic TCA. I use a mild to moderate glycolic acid or Jessner's peel on darker or sensitive complexions and find it produces more predictable results and is less irritating.

Someone who's looking to make long-term improvements to prevent aging would benefit more from fractional laser treatments. Mild to moderate peels improve what's on the surface but don't prevent future damage by thickening the dermis.

How long does it take? The peel itself takes approximately twenty to thirty minutes. Some peels are washed off after three minutes; TCA peels are applied and remain on the face since they neutralize automatically.

How does it feel? The sensation during a 30% TCA type of peel (which is moderate to more extreme) rises like a crescendo—like going up a roller coaster, getting to the top, then making a dramatic descent. The peel has a slow onset; then you begin to feel pinprick tingles, which intensify more and more into thousands of tiny, sharp stings for about six minutes until it gradually calms down. At its worst point, I've had people describe it as feeling like a hot curling iron hitting your face repeatedly. Most of my patients say that applying numbing cream for ten to fifteen minutes before the peel helps to minimize the pain. I also use a liquid nitrogen sweep, manually moving swabs of dry ice above the skin to cool it off.

Pain factor:
Lower-concentration glycolic or 10% TCA: ☹ to ☹
30% TCA and higher: ☹ ☹ ☹

Side effects and recovery: With a 30% TCA peel, the skin is lobster red for three or four days; then it becomes extremely dry and itchy; and finally it peels for about four days. I recommend that my patients come back for microdermabrasion one week later to remove any vestiges of dead skin that are left. After that the complexion is absolutely radiant.

A milder glycolic peel will leave small, dry, flaky areas, which will wash off in the shower.

Postprocedure pearls: Keep the skin moisturized with a super-thick emollient ointment. This forms a protective barrier that allows the skin to heal faster and also helps with scabbing. Do not pick at peeling skin. Never, ever, ever pick! This dead surface layer is retained by the body until it resurfaces itself. Pulling off skin that's still stuck is like pulling bark off a tree—it can damage what's underneath and leave a scar. You can use a soft, soapy, wet washcloth to gently massage the dead skin off.

After a peel, try to stay out of the sun completely for at least seven days. If you can't avoid being outside, try using a sunscreen made for babies or sensitive skin. It won't sting or irritate as much.

Social downtime: Even a light peel can mean two or three days of unpretty skin, while a 30% TCA means at least five to seven days of social lockdown. A deeper peel could involve up to three weeks since the entire top layer of the skin is burned away and the skin needs time to make a fresh new surface. There's no reason not to go to work during the red or peeling stages (it doesn't hurt), but you may get some strange looks and might have some explaining to do to your colleagues. (I worked every day after my peel and just told everyone the truth.)

When do you see results? After the side effects wear off, you will see glowing fresh skin revealed—usually about a week to ten days after a TCA peel.

How long do they last? After completing the series of peels recommended by your dermatologist, it's your new skin. If you protect it and maintain its health with sunscreen and moisturizer, the results can last for years.

Follow-up sessions: Most doctors recommend a series of five glycolic peels, while TCA peels require about three treatments to produce the desired result. With just one peel you'll see a big superficial difference, but a series will produce noticeably improved skin integrity because the repetition has a greater chance of spurring collagen production in the dermis. With glycolic peels, patients can come in once a month for five months. With TCA they can repeat the treatment every three months.

Lasers

What do they do? Different types of light or energy sources convert energy to heat in (or on) the skin in order to effect some kind of change: decimating brown spots or red spider veins, firming the skin, resurfacing it, and even building up collagen and elastin. Like different types of peels and fillers, each modality is made to target a specific skin condition, and some work better than others for certain antiaging issues or on various skin types. Fractionated laser, for example, is the best for building collagen and elastin and producing long-term antiaging results as well as resurfacing the skin. Intense pulsed light (IPL) is not as aggressive as fractionated laser and won't supply the same kind of serious antiaging benefits (although there are some), but it works well for discoloration and rosacea and has the upside of very little downtime and a lot less pain. Q-switched lasers zone in on pigment and vascular beam lasers are used on redness (discussed in chapter 8) and for removing tattoo ink from the dermis too. Radio-frequency devices work to firm the skin by heating the deep layers of tissue beneath the dermis, making them contract to firm the skin.

How do they work? All these devices deliver heat to the skin by way of an energy source, through different variations of light or radio frequency. Lasers work with a monochromatic wavelength of light generated by liquid dye, crystals (like ruby or alexandrite), metal (a semiconductor like a diode), or gases (like CO_2). IPL utilizes polychromatic light—a spectrum of wavelengths instead of one pure beam. IPL is something of a jack-of-all-trades light source that can address several skin issues at once, while monochromatic laser systems can be more dependable at treating a specific problem (for instance, using the Nd:YAG for brown spots).

There are three parameters a dermatologist can adjust on most lasers. The first is the pulse duration, or how long the energy is delivered to the skin. Longer pulse durations are necessary, and safer, for darker skin types, for example. They give the epidermis time to cool off and dissipate the thermal energy, so the skin doesn't burn. The second is the energy setting, which is measured in joules, and the third is the spot size, which corresponds to the diameter of the light beam that's coming out. The name of each laser specifies what wavelength it uses. For instance, I can say, "I'm going to use the 585 nanometer," or I'd refer to it as a pulsed dye laser.

For antiaging in general, a doctor uses resurfacing lasers. In the past, these were ablative techniques, meaning the lasers (either a CO_2 resurfacing laser or an erbium: YAG) physically broke through the epidermis and into the dermis. This laser destroys almost everything in its path, creating a controlled wound that sets off a healing response in the skin, rebuilding the extracellular matrix and resurfacing the raw top of the skin. This is the most invasive, extreme laser procedure, and CO_2 resurfacing usually requires general anesthesia. The recovery time for ablative laser resurfacing is almost three months, and the process can be grueling and painful. For most cosmetic dermatologists, this has been replaced by fractionated laser resurfacing, a hybrid between ablative and nonablative. This is much less painful, although it still hurts quite a bit, and the downtime is considerably less, about a week. Instead of scorching the entire surface of the skin with one beam, this laser drills microthermal holes into it using hundreds of coherent, but separate, beams. This leaves minute spaces of untouched skin interspersed amid these microscopic pinholes. Imagine the skin as a pegboard or latticework pattern, where a fraction of the skin is targeted each time. There are fractional erbium:YAG lasers (the type I use in my office) and fractional CO_2 lasers, which are much more intense. The fractionated technique doesn't leave the face decimated, just temporarily red, but it still creates the controlled wound that sets the reconstruction of the skin into motion.

Radio-frequency devices are nonablative, in that they do not affect the surface of the skin, so there's no real downtime or redness. They deliver heat via electromagnetic energy into the deep, fibrous tissue and fat beneath the dermis, causing it to contract and shrink permanently. The results of this technique are unpredictable, but it works well for some.

>>> TYPES OF LASER TREATMENT

These are the primary tools in the laser category that are used to address the aspects of antiaging. This guide will make it easier to keep them straight and help you sort out the pros and cons of each. There are many more device names available in each modality.

MODALITY	DEVICE NAMES	BEST FOR	PAIN FACTOR	RECOVERY TIME
Ablative	erbium:YAG, CO_2	Radical resurfacing of the skin and rebuilding of the extracellular matrix	☹☹ ☹☹+	Approximately 3 months
Non-ablative	Smoothbeam, CoolTouch (midinfrared lasers)	The first lasers proven to increase collagen production (now all lasers do and these are almost obsolete)	☹ to ☹☹	1–6 hours

MODALITY	DEVICE NAMES	BEST FOR	PAIN FACTOR	RECOVERY TIME
Fractionated resurfacing laser	Fraxel, Affirm	Antiaging (prevention, collagen building), resurfacing and exfoliating skin, firming lax skin	☹☹ ☹☹	2–7 days
Intense pulsed light	IPL	Poikiloderma (brown, white, red sun damage), rosacea, antiaging	☹ to ☹☹	1–3 hours
Pigment lasers	Q-switched Nd:YAG, ruby, Vbeam	Brown spots (Nd:YAG), spider veins (Ruby or Vbeam)	☹ to ☹☹	3 days– 3 weeks
Radio frequency	Thermage, Aluma	Moderate tightening of lax skin (like the jowls and neck)	☹☹ ☹☹ (for Thermage)	0–1 day
Infrared	Titan	Slight tightening of lax skin (doesn't go deeper than the dermis; results are unpredictable)	☹☹ ☹☹ (at high levels)	0–1 day

Who should try it? See the table above.

Who should not? Dark skin types (Fitzpatrick Types 5 and 6) should stay away from IPL and pigment-targeting lasers such as the Nd:YAG, since they can cause postinflammatory hypo- or hyperpigmentation (PIH). An exception to this rule: certain birthmarks around the eye and on the back, called "the nevus of Ito and Ota" respectively, are more common in darker skin types and are treated with the Nd:YAG laser. There's no way to adjust the pulse duration on most IPL devices, so it gives off a lot of energy to the epidermis (which in turn can trigger pigmentation problems in dark skin). Fractionated laser has been proven safe for all skin types in the hands of a knowledgeable MD.

How long does it take?

Fractionated laser: Ten to forty minutes (plus one hour of wearing a lidocaine numbing mask previous to the procedure).

Pigment laser: A few minutes to target the lesion or vessel and zap it.

IPL: Twenty to thirty minutes.

Radio frequency: This takes longer than most laser treatments—up to one hour, not including the topical anesthesia.

How does it feel?

Fractionated laser: Even after an hour of numbing cream, this procedure hurts. Some patients describe it as feeling like "hot needles sticking deep into the skin," and I can vouch for the fact that it's a deep, hot, sharp pain. (For most people, it's much more intense than a 30% TCA chemical peel). But many patients are surprisingly comfortable, even at the highest settings.

Pigment laser: This feels like a sharp, hot snap as the laser vaporizes the target spot.

IPL: The tip of the device feels cold against your skin; then, when it's fired, there's a bright light (like a camera flash) in your face and a hot rubber-band snap to accompany each flash. Like with any laser device, I can dial the joules down (or up) to decrease (or increase) the energy level, which adjusts the pain level as well. Though we offer numbing cream, most patients don't find it necessary.

Radio frequency: I had this done once on an area of skin, just to feel it. (Okay, I confess—also to tighten my early jowls!) I used a numbing cream for thirty minutes, and I had to stop the procedure because it was too much for me. It feels like a hot poker pushing into your skin on and off, over and over. Maybe next time I'll take a Valium, too.

Pain factor: See the table on pages 332–333.

Side effects and recovery:

Fractionated laser: The skin is red and warm (it looks and feels as if you have a sunburn), and there is some swelling for approximately thirty-six hours. For people with sensitive skin, I recommend taking an antihistamine before and after the procedure to decrease inflammation. Oral steroids can also help reduce the swelling of any treatment. On day 3 or 4 your skin appears slightly bronzed and feels rough because all those pixel-like pinholes are releasing crusting specks of dead skin.

Pigment laser: Brown spots or spider veins both look worse before they get better. They've been blown up by laser heat, so a brown spot becomes a dark maroon splotch until it flakes off in three to twenty-one days.

IPL: There are slight redness and swelling for one to three hours. On the chest, a bronzing effect can last a few weeks due to hemosiderin (pigment from the breakdown of blood vessels).

Radiofrequency: There could be slight swelling or redness, although some people have few visible side effects and no pain whatsoever once the treatment is finished.

Postprocedure pearls:

For all laser procedures: Keep the skin moist with an emollient wound-healing ointment. When the skin begins to flake, use a wet washcloth with lotion to massage it off. No fancy creams, and no sun exposure for one week.

Social downtime: See table on pages 332–333.

When do you see results?

Fractionated laser: After seven days. But it may take four to five treatments to achieve optimal results (on average, within six months).

Pigment laser: Three to ten days, depending on the body site being treated. Brown spots on legs and arms can take longer to go away than those on the face, which usually take three days to disappear. Legs can take months.

IPL: After the second or third treatment you notice decreased redness, freckles, and fine lines, and the skin has a smoother texture.

How long do they last? With all laser treatments, the results are forever. Depending on your biology, genetics, and good maintenance habits, the results last until your body ages naturally.

Follow-up sessions:

Fractionated laser: I usually recommend a series of three to five treatments.

Pigment laser: Often just one treatment does the trick, but if not a second one will. I always advise one to three treatments.

IPL: For the longest-lasting results, I suggest between five and twelve treatments. Since there's little downtime, the procedure can be repeated weekly.

Radio frequency: Usually a series of one to three is recommended since it has a cumulative effect.

>>> q&a

Q: I've heard that IPL and lasers can cause changes in skin cells. Is it safe to undergo this procedure if I had early-stage in situ melanoma removed years ago?

A: There is currently no evidence that lasers or intense pulsed light devices cause DNA changes to skin cells, and there have been no reports of this happening in the decade that they have been in use. Adequate safety studies have been done on these devices, and they've been proven safe. At Mount Sinai we did an in vivo study to see if pigment lasers (Q-switched Nd:YAG) could change the DNA or cause mutations in skin cells. Preexisting brown spots (benign nevi and lentigines, or freckles) were lasered and later tested to see if they were converted into cancerous lesions. We found no signs of mutation after biopsying the areas. (In fact, the ruby laser is a proven treatment for in situ melanoma, as augmentation to excision.) I would feel safe treating your skin with IPL or any other laser.

Q: Are the new at-home lasers effective? Are they safe to use?

A: Most of these over-the-counter gadgets are approved for safety by the FDA, and therefore their strength is limited. But even though they give off low-level energy, I worry about adverse effects that might happen on the wrong skin type if the instructions aren't followed at home. (Darker skin types should never use these things, since even though they emit low doses of light, they can cause postinflammatory hyperpigmentation.) Most of these contraptions aren't really "lasers" at all but LED (light-emitting diode) devices that use light to supposedly boost collagen and somehow improve the complexion. I'm not a big believer in the medical-grade LED machines used in doctor's offices (a panel of lights that a person sits in front of for a few minutes), so I'm doubtful about how much a handheld home LED can accomplish.

A new at-home IPL device has just received FDA clearance.

Though the FDA requires this particular machine to be sold in a doctor's office as a safety precaution and it puts out a fraction of the energy that a doctor's office machine emits, I still question its safety for use at home. For the most part, these thermal devices can be a good way to complement an office procedure, but they have limitations for much else. Home gadgets for treating acne and for hair removal may work well enough to be modestly helpful for maintenance, but they aren't going to provide much in the way of real results. Since these do-it-yourself machines are expensive ($1,000 to $2,000) and offer only mild payoffs, it's probably more worthwhile to get the job done professionally, reliably, and safely at a doctor's office. However, new promising handheld devices are becoming available at affordable prices.

Botox and Dysport (and new neurotoxins)

What does it do? Injections of botulinum toxin type A is the number one cosmetic procedure in the world, with more than 4 million treatments done in the United States in 2006. (Interestingly, 60 percent of female Botox users have never had any cosmetic surgery before, according to the Aesthetic Surgery Education and Research Foundation.) Its supreme popularity is for a good reason: it works. Botox and Dysport are purified forms of botulinum toxin type A (and no, the shots do not produce the deadly disease botulism). When injected in tiny amounts, the neurotoxin causes facial muscles to relax and almost magically erases frown lines, forehead wrinkles, and crow's feet. Because it smoothes the skin, the procedure also makes slight structural changes to the face: opening up the eyes, widening the forehead, and elevating the brows. There are more than forty muscles in the face, and they all interconnect and work together. Some are elevators (lifting up), and some are depressors (moving downward). With this neurotoxin, if you inject one muscle that elevates, you might get a drop in another muscle. To counteract that drop, you need to inject the drug into a depressor muscle to get an elevation. The doctor must know how to balance out one injection with another. More than any other procedure, Botox or Dysport injections require a good understanding of how the muscle fibers interconnect with one another.

The first real competitor to the Botox throne, Dysport (abobotulinumtoxin A), formerly known as Reloxin, works similarly and is now FDA-approved for cosmetic purposes. With the immense success of Botox, new forms of muscle-relaxing drugs and devices that target nerve receptors are evolving and being developed constantly.

How does it work? For aesthetic work, Botox and Dysport are used in almost homeopathic doses, very tiny amounts. They both block the nerve receptors on the muscle, paralyzing the ones that cause actions that reinforce wrinkles such as crow's feet, marionette lines, and forehead furrows. Think of the receptor as a baseball mitt and Botox or Dysport as the ball. Once it lodges itself in that receptor nothing else can get in, so it blocks any signals that would trigger the muscle to move. Receptors (like skin cells) have a limited life span, and they are constantly being renewed. A blocked receptor is blocked until it dies off and a new receptor takes its place. This is why the effects of Botox and Dysport are temporary and muscle movement returns. Once the drug sticks in the receptor, it stays there like a key in a lock and does not travel or function anywhere else.

Who should try it? Anyone who is bothered by fine lines or wrinkles is a perfect candidate, but botulinum toxins have other off-label uses. They've been shown to be a good treatment for migraine headaches and also block receptors in the sweat glands (so shots under the arm decrease perspiration). Many dermatologists use this drug to manipulate the shape of the face slightly too. A touch of Botox at the base of the nose gives it a more turned-up appearance, and an injection at the upper lip can bring it down slightly and minimize a gummy smile.

Who should not? Botulinum toxins work wonders on lines and wrinkles, but they do nothing for sun damage or skin texture. For those issues, I suggest laser treatments or chemical peels. Botox has been tested thoroughly since the FDA approved it for cosmetic use in 2002 and has been proven safe. Recently, an Italian medical study done on mice found that botulinum neurotoxins migrated to their brains.[1] Doctors read through the literature and were not worried about the ramifications, since any safe medication will be harmful to a small animal if it's overdosed with it. The study was interesting but not clinically relevant to cosmetic use in humans because the dosage is very small and the risk of migration is extremely low. It was certainly taken seriously, and there is a black box label warning, but the judgment remains that Botox and Dysport are safe for cosmetic use.

Patients with certain neuromuscular diseases (such as multiple sclerosis) or autoimmune diseases (such as lupus) need clearance from their specialist before considering any injectable.

How long does it take? The injections generally take five to ten minutes but may take up to thirty minutes.

How does it feel? Like sharp pinpricks. Most of my patients don't even ask for numbing cream (they're old hands after the first treatment), and there's no real need for it. I think for most people it's the needle phobia that scares them.

Pain factor: 🙁

Side effects and recovery: The most common side effect is some slight bruising at the site of the injections, and (rarely) some people develop a headache afterward. A more serious complication of Botox injections can be ptosis, when the eyebrow and eyelid droop. This can happen when the skin is too lax or when the muscles right above the brow or the ones between them are injected. Often a slight one- or two-millimeter drop reverses within two weeks, but unfortunately the effect can last as long as the Botox results and there's no way to reverse it. There's a long list of potential side effects you should be aware of before consenting to this procedure, but most of them are extremely rare. Check the official web sites (botoxcosmetic.com or www.dysport.co.nz) for more information.

Social downtime: None.

When do you see results? Usually in four to seven days or up to two weeks.

How long do they last? Three to nine months.

Postprocedure pearls: To minimize the bruising that occurs with any procedure, especially those involving needles, many of my patients swear by the herbal remedy *Arnica montana*. Topical creams and tinctures can be applied on the bruise itself, and taking homeopathic arnica tablets before and after the treatment is believed to decrease trauma to the skin. Eating foods containing vitamin K, such as spinach and broccoli, may help blood coagulate and reduce bruising too (although applying it topically is ineffectual). Don't take a nap or press on the area for eight hours because you may push the neurotoxin to a different muscle and develop ptosis. The last thing you'd want to do is have any kind of facial massage afterward. I don't like to do fractionated laser and Botox on the same day, for instance, because the patient gets swelling from the laser procedure and that can make the neurotoxin migrate.

Follow-up sessions: Follow-up appointments one to two weeks after the initial procedure are the key to preventing an overly injected, frozen look. This is especially important for first-time Botox or Dysport patients, since I prefer to err on the side of using fewer units initially and leaving the face with some natural expression and muscle movement. I know I can always touch up and add more if the patient wants it, but once it's been injected the muscles are paralyzed for months. Experienced dermatologists are aware of the ptosis possibilities and stay away from those muscles, which is another good reason to have Botox done only by an experienced medical professional.

>>> q&a

Q: If you stop Botox or Dysport, will the lines get worse? Is it preventative?

A: The lines don't get worse because Botox has immobilized them. But once it wears off, you go back to baseline—back to the lines you already had, to your own reality. The disturbing, Dorian Gray–like experience of seeing those lines and wrinkles return seems to happen overnight. This is why, for many women, the treatment becomes an act of routine beauty maintenance. Relaxing one muscle may cause some people to begin using other muscles in their face to compensate for the ones that are paralyzed. If you seem to notice new lines, go in for a touch-up. Because Botox and Dysport stop dynamic muscle contractions that create creases and furrows, the treatment can be relatively preventive. If you stop doing Botox, you go back to making the muscle movements that gave you some of those lines. Repeated treatments do cause the muscles to atrophy, which naturally weakens them and suppresses their movement. For this reason, the trend among young girls in their twenties wanting to have Botox as a preventive measure is disturbing. While I won't discriminate if a young person has obvious lines and wrinkles he or she wants softened, I will not administer Botox or Dysport to a young girl who doesn't need it (and neither will any other ethical dermatologist).

Injectable Fillers

What do they do? Dermal fillers deliver volume and youthful plumpness to a sinking or flat section of the skin instantly. (Imagine refilling a lumpy, flat down pillow with fresh, fluffy feathers.) They can fill shadowy hollows under the eyes, plump up falling nasolabial folds (the creases from both sides of the nose to the outer corners of the mouth), or fill in sagging marionette lines near the mouth.

This is such a breakthrough territory in cosmetic dermatology, and with the evolving quality and diversity of these fillers combined with developing techniques for their use, we can practically provide a face-lift using various fillers strategically injected. The cheek area becomes flatter with age, and filling in the apples of the cheeks can lend a rounder, softer appearance and make the face look younger. Restoring volume changes the tension vectors in the face, so it can lift an area (such as the cheekbone or temples) slightly. Placed at the right spots on a bumpy nose, filler can even make it straighter (nonsurgical rhinoplasty). I can elongate a weak chin with filler or strengthen the jawline (and consequently decrease the appearance of jowls) by injecting it at the base of the jaw near the ear. It's all about balancing the shape of the face.

The big bonus is that most fillers are scientifically proven to build collagen in the dermis. They are considered "semi-permanent" for this reason, since when the filler wears off, new collagen has replaced some of it. I worked on a study that found that calcium hydroxylapatite (Radiesse) did just that.[2] Most fillers are essentially tiny beads that are cross-linked together and suspended in a gel vehicle. Once injected, the gel dissipates and the cross-linked microspheres act as a scaffolding structure around which your own body forms collagen, until those beads eventually disintegrate too. How cool is that? On top of that, the deep injection itself can create a controlled wound-healing response. It's been found that successive refill treatments require less filler because new collagen has been produced to fill up the area.

How do they work? As crazy as it sounds, injecting dermal filler into different levels of the dermis is similar to filling a jelly doughnut, in that a hole is pierced into a pressurized system. The extracellular matrix is the dough that holds the filler in place. Fillers are derived from four sources. Synthetic materials are silicone, calcium hydroxylapatite, poly-L-lactic acid, and polymethylmethacrylate (PMMA). These are the heavyweights, not just because of their permanent or semipermanent aspect but because they can be very dense, like calcium hydroxylapatite, or offer high volume, like poly-L-lactic acid (Sculptra). Sculptra is a solution—(more watery than other gel fillers)—that provides a great fill effect on a large area, but the downside is that the extra fluid dissipates quickly and requires refilling every three to five months for three to five treatments until it builds up and stimulates the body to build its own collagen.

Collagen fillers are either taken from cows or pigs or bioengineered from human tissue. Hyaluronic acid fillers are derivations of the same water-binding substance that's found in our bodies and hydrates the skin. The fourth alternative involves harvesting your own fat through liposuction, purifying it, and injecting it into the face. Though the results can be permanent in many people and the more organic notion of recycling your own fat is positive, it requires an added, expensive and uncomfortable liposuction procedure.

What goes where, and why? Interestingly enough, the qualities of the ideal filler are different for doctors than they are for patients. From a doctor's perspective, we look for longevity, safety, a minimum of side effects, reliable results, cost-effectiveness, ease of injectability, biocompatibility, natural look, reversibility, and less pain. A patient wants a filler with (in order of importance), less pain, longevity, a natural look, reliable results, and minimal downtime. And low cost!

Every doctor has preferences about which filler to inject into which part of the face. These are based on everything from how the filler flows through the syringe (they all have differing viscosity levels) to how it feels or looks in a particular area of the face. Radiesse, for instance, has such heft and thickness that it provides ballast for strong areas such as the cheekbone, the jawbone, and the nasolabial folds. It's also great for men. For someone with fine features a doctor will probably use lighter, thinner fillers that are compatible with the patient's facial structure. Heavier, thicker ones in a delicate face can look like an artificial implant. Ask your dermatologist what he or she recommends. I would trust the doctor's ideas and opinions. The type of filler used varies with every patient. I make a master plan during the consultation, so the procedures are tailor-made for that individual patient. That being said, these are some of the most common fillers to target specific zones of the face and neck:

Temples (V-shaped lateral orbital circle): Sculptra or a hyaluronic acid filler is best.

Forehead: Collagen is wonderful for these fine lines.

Under the brow: A hyaluronic acid such as Restylane or Juvéderm can add some structure to the brow bone area.

Nose: Radiesse or hyaluronic acid, since they are easy to sculpt with and long-lasting.

Crow's feet: Collagen or hyaluronic acids is best.

Under the eyes: The delicate under-eye area needs a thinner, transparent hyaluronic acid filler such as Restylane or Juvéderm.

Earlobes: Yes, these too become droopy and wrinkled with age. I prefer to use hyaluronic acid filler to plump and restore structure to the lobes.

Nasolabial folds and marionette lines: This area can support a denser filler such as Radiesse, Perlane, or Juvéderm Ultra Plus. This area needs a lot of product to make a significant difference; finer fillers get lost in this "Bermuda Triangle" zone in the mid third of the face. Even high-volume Sculptra could work since so much is needed.

Cheeks and cheekbones: Sculptra or thicker hyaluronic acids such as Perlane or Radiesse.

Lips: Obviously, soft filler is preferable for lips. Collagen (which has less downtime but wears off faster) or a slightly firmer hyaluronic acid such as Restylane or Juvéderm is best.

Jaw line: A thicker filler such as Radiesse bolsters the mandibular angle near the ear and lifts the face.

Chin: Almost any type of filler works here.

Neck: To fill those horizontal lines, a hyaluronic acid like Restylane or Juvéderm is best. I've also had success with Radiesse and Sculptra in this area. (See Q&A on sagging necks)

Some great ideas for fillers.

>>> FILLERS

You probably thought laser choices were confusing until you arrived at this overwhelming array of fillers (and there are new ones on the horizon all the time). Just as the 1980s were the era of new laser systems, now is the age of new fillers. (I predict that there will soon be some that inspire fat to grow around them, in addition to collagen.) Use this guide when your dermatologist suggests different fillers for your particular concerns. Each filler is unique, and an experienced doctor knows which works best for a certain area or which might last longer in a particular spot.

The price of fillers varies among products and is dependent on the doctor, the area of the country where you have the procedure done, and so on. Fillers are expensive for a doctor to purchase, so a patient should expect to spend between $500 and $3,000. Another big variable is the length of time a filler lasts. Since many work to build collagen, the results can last longer than this timeline suggests. And the results vary from person to person.

FORM	FILLER NAMES	BEST FOR	LASTS FOR
Synthetic	Silicone Artefill Radiesse (calcium hydroxylapatite) Sculptra	Calcium-based Radiesse is thicker and works best in places like the nasolabial folds and marionette lines that are in a naturally fuller part of the face. Sculptra is a thinner solution that's injected, then molded into place under the skin. Great for larger areas like cheeks.	Silicone is permanent and rarely used these days by specialists. Artefill is permanent. Radiesse usually lasts 9 months–2 years. Sculptura (once it's been built up with 3–5 treatments) lasts about 1–2 years. Since it builds collagen, this timeline can be even longer.

FORM	FILLER NAMES	BEST FOR	LASTS FOR
Collagen	Cosmoplast Zyplast Zyderm Cosmoderm Evolance	Used for "spackling" or filling in super-fine lines around the mouth, eyes, or forehead.	Very temporary: 1–3 months. Evolance is longer lasting: 6–12 months.
Hyaluronic Acid	Restylane Juvéderm Juvéderm Ultra Plus Perlane	Juvéderm Ultra Plus and Perlane are denser fillers—but still soft.	Anywhere from 6 months to 2 years, depending on the individual and the area of the face.
Fat	Autologous fat transfer	Used on many areas on the face, neck, hands, and feet.	Can be permanent on some people, but fat can be resorbed on some and goes away over time.

Who should try it? Those who have dark circles associated with sunken eyes or a loss of volume anywhere—commonly in the nasolabial folds and marionette lines. Fillers can also restore a stronger shape and structure to the face by adding volume to sinking areas (like filling a deflated, shapeless inner tube with air).

Who should not? Fillers are not meant to tighten the skin per se, although adding volume will firm the skin slightly as a consequence. Filling up a flattened area may also soften lines as a result, but Botox is a better wrinkle eraser (I often do a combination of Botox and filler to take care of crow's feet and restore volume to the lateral orbital area).

Fillers have been proven safe for darker skin types and won't cause scarring or postinflammatory hyperpigmentation. I was the lead author of an FDA study that proved the safety of calcium hydroxylapatite injected into the nasolabial folds of persons of color.[3] Other similar studies have been performed with the HA's.

How long does it take? Depending on where an injection is placed, the patient usually has a topical numbing cream applied first and sometimes a lidocaine injection administered (especially for fillers in the nasolabial folds). The filler injections themselves usually take five to thirty minutes per area.

How does it feel? If you imagine how it feels to have a substance injected under your eyes or near your mouth, you'd be about right. It's unpleasant, and it does hurt—but probably not as much as you think it will. Some areas of the face (usually places where nerves and vessels are closer to the surface such as the marionette lines, the lips, and the apples of the cheeks) are more painful than others. Also, bigger, more viscous fillers, such as Radiesse and Perlane, stretch the skin, and this creates an extremely achy, throbbing feeling for about twenty minutes right after the injection. It usually is not painful after the procedure is finished, though.

Pain factor: ☹ ☹ to ☹ ☹ ☹

Side effects and recovery: You are guaranteed to get some degree of bruising and swelling where you were injected. There's usually more swelling with hyaluronic acid fillers, since they bind water in the skin, absorbing like a sponge on purpose. So for a few days you may look as if you've been in a bar fight.

Sometimes fillers can create bumpiness underneath the skin. That's why the dermatologist will gently press the area after filling it, to make sure it's smooth and even.

Social downtime: Bruises usually fade after five to ten days. Swelling should go down in about two or three days.

When do you see results? Immediately! I can see the shape of the face evolve, like watching a photograph develop. I even give the patient a mirror so he or she can see the effects and I can add a little more filler if they would like. (Remember, though, that some of the fullness and puffiness you will see in the next few days is due to swelling. The end result may not be fully apparent till that inflammation has gone down.)

How long do they last? See table on pages 346–347.

Postprocedure pearls: Again, topical or systemic *Arnica montana* can be helpful to diminish bruising. A cold ice pack will reduce any swelling. You can also elevate your head on a couple extra pillows when you sleep.

For hyaluronic acid fillers, there is a magic eraser called hyaluronidase. It's one of my favorite antidotes because it takes the risk out of using these fillers (it won't work on synthetic, fat, or collagen, however). Hyaluronidase is an enzyme that, when injected into an overfilled spot and massaged around the area, dissolves the filler, completely reversing the procedure.

Follow-up sessions: There are three fillers that require a series of treatments: Sculptra, which needs to be repeated until it builds up to a plateau level (since a large percentage of this watery solution dissipates into the skin). Fat requires up to five injections to achieve the ideal fill. Silicone requires the doctor to inject a lot of microdroplets under the skin, wait approximately one month for the silicone beads to settle, and then inject a bit more during another appointment until the desired effect is achieved.

>>> q&a
_____

Q: My hands look twenty years older than my face, with sunspots, crepey skin and ugly, visible veins. Can cosmetic procedures work beyond the face?

A: Absolutely! The skin ages the same way all over the body, and the hands (and feet) can benefit from the very same techniques that make a face look more youthful. They suffer from the same loss of fat, collagen, and elastin, so injecting filler can add a layer above the bones and veins, giving the hands a softer, fuller look. I like to use thicker, high-volume filler here because it's such a large area. Since it's more viscous and watery, Sculptra is easy to inject in between each finger at the tops of the hands and then mold into place like clay. But with Sculptra, this procedure needs to be repeated a few times because so much of it dissipates. Radiesse, Perlane, or Juvéderm Ultra Plus can be an ideal alternative, one that's longer-lasting and more convenient, since only one procedure is necessary to do the job.

A pigment-specific laser such as Nd:YAG can get rid of sunspots and brown spots on the backs of the hands. Once those spots have been lasered, they turn red and then dark before they flake off, so your hands can look much worse for one to two weeks before they look much better. I often do fractionated laser treatments on the hands and forearms. This evens out the tone and complexion of the skin and helps build collagen in the dermis after three to five treatments (the same amount that's recommended for the face). Hands, like all the skin below your face, are usually forgotten when it comes to sunscreen, which is why we have such extreme skin aging there. You will need to use a hand cream or body lotion with sun protection to prevent more sun damage in the future.

Q: Is there anything noninvasive that can really help my sagging neck, short of plastic surgery?

A: I hear this question a lot. (The title of Nora Ephron's book *I Feel Bad about My Neck* is such a refreshing and hilariously honest statement!) For those who feel bad about their necks, it becomes an obsession. It's the first thing you see when you look in the mirror, and until recently a neck lift was the best option available. Thankfully, there are many more noninvasive alternatives, although none of them will provide the dramatic and permanent results that plastic surgery can.

One reason why the neck may have lost more elasticity than your face is twofold: it's thinner, more delicate skin, and we sun optimists overlook applying sunscreen anywhere below the face—until the damage is done, of course. Mild to moderate laxity can be treated with fractionated laser resurfacing (which also multitasks by resurfacing and improving the texture and appearance of the epidermis) or radio-frequency procedures like Thermage to contract the deep tissue like a Shrinky Dink. These can be good alternatives for someone who's not ready for a face-lift and needs a minor amount of tightening. It's important to adjust your expectations of skin-firming techniques such as these, because they will make only a slight improvement. Again, this is not a surgical neck lift. To treat a double chin or jowls, cosmetic dermatologists and plastic surgeons use liposuction to eliminate the extra fat (although this may also increase skin laxity in the area). A filler injected at the jawbone—at the mandibular angle near the earlobe—can resculpt the jaw line and make it more angular, which in turn balances the face and diminishes jowls. To soften the horizontal lines on the neck, filler can be injected directly into them. Botox can be used on the muscles that drape underneath the jaw line to tuck it up a little bit, or can be injected into the vertical bands in the middle of the neck to relax and flatten out that muscle. Both of these solutions offer unpredictable results, and sometimes an entire bottle of Botox needs to be used in this area to effect any kind of change.

Q: Can fillers be used to make my lips look just a little fuller and still natural? And can anything be done for those little lines above the top lip?

A: In many areas, such as the eyes, neck, or the lips, a doctor has to come at it with a few different approaches. The problems you are seeing are caused by multiple factors—a breakdown of collagen in the lips, repeated muscle movements that create those fine lines above the lips—and each responds to a specialized treatment. The solution is a combination of therapies. I use just a trace amount of Botox to relax the muscles creating dynamic wrinkling above the top lip, and a superficial filler like collagen can fill in those fine lines beautifully. To fill the lip and reassert a more defined border around it, I use soft hyaluronic acid filler. To avoid an overly inflated look, I usually suggest using less and following up within one to two weeks to add more filler if necessary. Or a collagen filler is very soft and natural and won't incur much swelling at all; it just doesn't last as long.

Often there is a lot of visible sun damage above the upper lip, and some people start to see solar elastosis (loss of the extracellular matrix that gives a slightly bumpy, cobblestone-like texture to the skin) there. This is an important place to do rejuvenation with a fractionated laser to even the skin tone and build up the extracellular matrix (and it's more cost-effective to do the laser procedure over the entire face and neck rather than in one small area of the face).

Conclusion

While reading this book, you have virtually spent a week or two with me in my practice. You've learned about everything from skin cancers to Botox injections. Together, we have explored health concerns, beauty enhancements, the key products you need to use on your skin, and the ones you don't need to bother with at all.

I'm a problem solver, and now you will be too. You can look at your skin and diagnose yourself, you know what to be concerned about and what shouldn't worry you, and you're aware of the straightforward and effective solutions out there. Armed with a better understanding of how your skin works and what it needs to stay healthy and beautiful, you now have greater confidence about how to care for it. Needless to say, you are something of a skin care expert at this point. You probably know more than most of the people selling you products do, and you may even know a little more about cosmetic ingredients than your own dermatologist does. I realize, and completely empathize, with your confusion at the beauty counter and with your health concerns. The aim of this book is to educate and, by doing so, offer reassurance about all of your skin questions and concerns (even the embarrassing ones). Once you understand the facts, taking care of your skin really is relatively simple.

I've found that many of my patients will point out a suspicious spot on their friend's or a family member's skin and urge that person to get it checked out. I've taught them what to look for, and they are more attentive and alert to skin changes as a result. Now you can watch out for your family, your partner, and your friends by noticing something that they may not. I encourage you to share this newfound knowledge with other people and—maybe you'll protect someone else or even save a life. I see this all the time.

It all comes back to my philosophy that you have more important and fun things to do than obsess about your complexion. Most of us have enough responsibilities to deal with. We don't need to be distracted by the pressure to have perfect movie star skin (which doesn't exist in real life, trust me) or to miraculously look like a twenty-year-old at the age of forty-eight. (Although, as you learned in chapter 10, there are wonderful ways to appear more youthful and rejuvenated and still look natural.) It's not impossible to have a beautiful complexion or even to look a little younger and more refreshed. It just shouldn't be your full-time job. It's mine.

Use this book as your guide and refer to it when you, or someone in your family, has a skin problem, when you are considering a cosmetic procedure, or if you need a refresher on what's in that miracle antiaging cream you are about to buy. I hope I've eliminated the intimidation involved with shopping for cosmetics. And you can draw on this book as a second opinion before you undergo a procedure. Again, knowing the facts gives you the ability to take charge. Wanting to look attractive (your personal best) is a healthy aspiration, and this psychology of beauty is powerful, but it has to be personal. The products you select should be what your skin needs (or an indulgence you desire), rather than something you are pushed into purchasing by the media or a salesperson. When in doubt, stick with the basics: cleanser, moisturizer, sunscreen. Keep it simple.

Acknowledgments

It takes a village to write a book, and this one is full of fantastic people. I have personally thanked many of them who helped along the way but wish to address a few pivotal people.

Thank you to the world-class team at Atria Books. To Judith Curr, an ingenious leader and publisher. It has been my great fortune to work with you. To the wonderful Greer Hendricks and Sarah Walsh, editors who made this book a thousand times more eloquent. Thanks to Jeanne Lee, Amy Saidens, Alysha Bullock, Jaime Putorti, Kim Curtin, and Kathleen Schmidt.

To Robin Straus, the perfect agent! Thank you for your guidance and friendship. To the smart, lovely, hilarious, and eloquent Gina Way, co-authoring this book with you was unbelievably fun. You made the hard parts easy and the easy parts intriguing. My eternal gratitude and friendship.

Thank you to my family, friends, staff, and mentors—Jonathan, Jonah, Julien, Sasha, Ezra, Nafi, Oumi, Aisha, Ben, Ann, John, Betty, John, Scott, Emmy, Alanna, Ching, Tani, Judy, Arlene, Paula, Gisselle, Dr. Lebwohl, Dr. Gordon, Dr. Waldorf, Dr. Turner, Dr. Franz, Dr. Phelps, Dr. Goldberg, Peter Hurley, Yves Durif, Connie, Charlene, Anna, and Robin. Thank you to the talented writer Jen Shotz who wrote the first SSB book proposal and to Milly Marmur, the famous book agent and my aunt-in-law. Finally, I am indebted to my patients—many of whom are authors—for your thoughts, enthusiasm, and insights that inspired this book.

—*Ellen Marmur, MD*

Thanks to the entire team at Atria Books—especially Judith Curr, Greer Hendricks, and Sarah Walsh—and to Robin Straus, for making this book a reality and such a satisfying experience. I'm indebted to Jaime Wolf, my attorney and protector, who somehow manages to make negotiations and legal business enjoyable. I'm grateful to my father, Don Way, for passing on his endless curiosity and his way with words to me, and to my beautiful mother, Joyce Way, for handing down some of her serenity and her perfect complexion. Special thanks to my husband, Benjamin Sontheimer, for his continuous support and belief in me. I'm also grateful to my friend Jodi Zimmerman, for insistently recommending that I make an appointment with her brilliant dermatologist: Dr. Ellen Marmur. And finally, to Ellen, you have been an extraordinary collaborator and have become a generous, trusted friend. Thank you for choosing me to help make your dream a reality, and for this challenging, fun, hilarious, fascinating journey together.

—*Gina Way*

Notes

CHAPTER 3 **FACTORS THAT INFLUENCE YOUR SKIN**

1. Glenda Hall and Tania J. Phillips, "Estrogen and Skin: The Effects of Estrogen, Menopause, and Hormone Replacement Therapy on the Skin," *Journal of the American Academy of Dermatology* 53, no. 4 (October 2005): 569–571.

2. Christiane Guinot et al., "Effect of Hormonal Replacement Therapy on Skin Biophysical Properties of Menopausal Women," *Skin Research and Technology* 11, no. 4 (October 12, 2005): 201–204.

3. M. G. Shah and H. I., "Estrogen and Skin. An Overview," *American Journal of Clinical Dermatology* 2, no. 3 (2001): 143–150.

4. Maeve Cosgrove et al., "Dietary Nutrient Intakes and Skin-aging Appearance Among Middle-aged American Women," *The American Journal of Clinical Nutrition* 86, no. 4 (October 2007): 1225–1231.

5. H. Wei, X. Zhang, J. F. Zhao, Z. Y. Wang, D. Bickers, and M. Lebwohl, *Free Radical Biology and Medicine* 26, nos. 11–12 (June 1999): 1427–1435.

6. A. Pappas, M. Anthonavage, and J. Gordon, "Metabolic Fate and Selective Utilization of Major Fatty Acids in Human Sebaceous Gland," *Journal of Investigative Dermatology* 118, no. 1 (January 2002): 164–171.

7. F. William Danby, "Acne and Milk, the Diet Myth, and Beyond," *Journal of American Academy of Dermatology* 52, no. 2 (February 2005): 360–362

8. RN Smith et al., "The Effect of a High-Protein, Low Glycemic-Load Diet Versus a Conventional, High Glycemic-load Diet on Biochemical Parameters Associated with Acne Vulgaris: A Randomized, Investigator-masked, Controlled Trial," *Journal of the American Academy of Dermatology* 57, no. 5 (2007): 247–256.

9. Arathi R. Setty, Gary Curhan, and Hyon K Choi, "Obesity, Waist Circumference, Weight Change, and the Risk of Psoriasis in Women," *Archives of Internal Medicine* 167, no. 15 (2007): 1670–1675.

10. Margaret Altemus et al., "Stress-induced Changes in Skin Barrier Function in Healthy Women," *Journal of Investigative Dermatology*, no. 2, 117 (August 2007): 309–317.

11. J. K. Kiecolt-Glaser et al., "Slowing of Wound Healing by Psychological Stress," *The Lancet* 346, no. 8984 (November 1995): 1194–1196.

12. F. Tausk et al., "Stressed Mice Quicker to get Skin Cancer," *Journal of the American Academy of Dermatology* 51, no. 6 (December 2004): 919–922.

13. A. Chiu, S. Y. Chon, and A. B. Kimball, "The Response of Skin Disease to Stress: Changes in the Severity of *Acne Vulgaris* as Affected by Examination Stress," *Archives of Dermatology* 139, no. 7 (July 2003) 2003: 897–900.

14. E. Epel, *Proceedings of the National Academy of Sciences*, Nov. 30, 2004, News Release, University of California, San Francisco.

15. A. Lowell Goldsmith, "Skin Effects of Air Pollution." *Otolaryngology—Head and Neck Surgery* 114, no. 2 (February 1996): 217–219.

16. A. Knuutinen, N. Kokkonen, J. Risteli, K. Vähäkangas, M. Kallioinen, T. Salo, T. Sorsa, and A. Oikarinen, "Smoking Affects Collagen Synthesis and Extracellular Matrix Turnover in Human Skin," *British Journal of Dermatology* 146, no. 4 (2002): 588–594.

CHAPTER 4 YOUR SERIOUSLY SIMPLE SKIN CARE PLAN

1. D. Ariely et al., "Commercial Features of Placebo and Therapeutic Efficacy," *The Journal of the American Medical Association* 299, no. 9 (March 5, 2008): 1016–1017.

CHAPTER 5 YOUR UV PROTECTION STRATEGY: ON THE BEACH, AT THE POOL, IN THE SUN ANYWHERE

1. Erica S. Hamant and Brian B. Adams, "Sunscreen Use Among Collegiate Athletes," *Journal of the American Academy of Dermatology* 53, no. 2 (August 2005): 237–241.

2. Philippe Autier et al., "Sunscreen Use and Duration of Sun Exposure: A Double-Blind, Randomized Trial," *Journal of the National Cancer Institute* 91, no. 15 (August 4, 1999): 1304–1309.

3. M. R. Karagas et al., "Use of Tanning Devices and Risk of Basal Cell and Squamous Cell Carcinomas," *Journal of the National Cancer Institute* 94, no. 3 (February 6, 2002): 224–226.

4. Marianne Placzek et al., "Ultraviolet B-Induced DNA Damage in Human Epidermis Is Modified by the Antioxidants Ascorbic Acid and Tocopherol," *Journal of Investigative Dermatology* 124, no. 2 (February 2005): 304–307.

5. D. H. McDaniel et al., "Idebenone: A New Antioxidant–Part 1. Relative Assessment of Oxidative Stress Protection Capacity Compared to Commonly Known Antioxidants." *Journal of Cosmetic Dermatology* 4, no. 1 (January 2005): 10–17.

6. S. Gonzalez et al., "Orally Administered Polypodium Leucotomos Extract Decreases Psoralen–UVA-induced Phototoxicity, Pigmentation, and Damage of Human Skin," *Journal of the American Academy of Dermatology* 51, no. 6 (December 2004): 910–918.

7. S. Gonzalez et al., "Topical or Oral Administration with an Extract of Polypodium Leucotomos Prevents Acute Sunburn and Psoralen-induced Phototoxic Reactions as well as Depletion of Langerhans Cells in Human Skin," *Photodermatology Photoimmunology Photomedicine* 13 nos. 1–2 (February–April 1997): 50–60.

8. Serge Hercberg et al., "Antioxidant Supplementation Increases the Risk of Skin Cancers in Women but not in Men," *The Journal of Nutrition* 137 (September 2007): 2098–2105.

9. R. B. Sollitto et al., "Normal Vitamin D Levels Can Be Maintained Despite Rigorous Photoprotection," *Journal of the American Academy of Dermatology* 37, no. 6 (December 1997): 942–947.

CHAPTER 7 SKIN CANCER

1. A Bleyer, M. O'Leary, R. Barr, L. A. G. Ries (eds.): "Cancer Epidemiology in Older Adolescents and Young Adults 15 to 29 Years of Age, Including SEER Incidence and Survival: 1975–2000," *National Cancer Institute*, NIH Pub. No. 06-5767, 2006.

2. H. Kittler, H. Pehanberger, K. Wolff, M. Binder, "Follow-up of Melanocytic Skin Lesions with Digital ELM: Patterns of Modifications Observed in Early Melanoma, Atypical Nevi, and Common Nevi," *Journal of the American Academy of Dermatology* 43, no. 3 (September 2000): 467–476.

3. A. Fuchs, E. Marmur, "The Kinetics of Skin Cancer: Progression of Actinic Keratosis to Squamous Cell Carcinoma," *Dermatologic Surgery* 33, no. 9 (September 2007): 1099–1101.

4. C. Yee, N. Hunder, L. Weiner, et al., "Treatment of Metastatic Melanoma with Autologous CD4+T Cells Against NY-ESO-1," *The New England Journal of Medicine* 358, no. 25 (June 2008): 2698–2703.

5. J. Xie et al., "Inhibition of Smoothened Signaling Prevents Ultraviolet B-Induced Basal Cell Carcinomas Through Regulation of Fas Expression and Apoptosis," *Cancer Research* 64, no. 20 (October 2004): 7545–7552.

CHAPTER 8 SKIN SOS: PROBLEMS AND PRESCRIPTIONS

1. D. J. Goldberg, E. S. Marmur, C. Schmults, M. Hussain, R. Phelps, "Histologic and Ultrastructural Analysis of Ultraviolet B Laser and Light Source Treatment of Leukoderma in Striae Distensae," *Dermatologic Surgery* 31, no. 4 (April 2005): 385–387.

2. M. S. Lolis, E. S. Marmur, "Paradoxical Effects of Hair Removal Systems: A Review," *Journal of Cosmetic Dermatology* 5, no. 4 (December 2006): 274–276.

CHAPTER 9 CRACKING THE CODE ON COSMECEUTICALS: CAN ANTIAGING PRODUCTS MAKE US LOOK YOUNGER, AND WHICH ONES REALLY WORK?

1. Eugene A. Bauer et al., "Retinoic Acid Inhibition of Collegenase and Gelatinase Expression in Human Skin Fibroblast Cultures. Evidence for a Duel Mechanism," *Journal of Investigative Dermatology* 81, no. 2 (August 1983): 162–169.

2. D. Feskanich, V. Singh, et al., "Vitamin A Intake and Hip Fractures Among Postmenopausal Women," *Journal of the American Medical Association,* 287 no 1 (January 2002): 47–54.

3. H. Melhus et al., "Excessive Dietary Intake of Vitamin A is Associated with Reduced Bone Mineral Density and Increased Risk of Hip Fracture," *Annals of Internal Medicine* 120, no. 10 (November 1998): 770–778.

4. A. B. Kimball, D. L. Bissett, L. R. Robinson, J. Li, K. Miyamoto, T. L. Grosick, et al., "Topical Formulation Containing N-acetyl Glucosamine and Niacinamide Reduces the Appearance of Photoaging on Human Facial Skin (abstract)," *Journal of the American Academy of Dermatology* 54, no. 3 (2006): AB43.

5. R. Osborne, L. Mullins, et al., "Topical N-acetyl Glucosamine and Niacinamide Increase Hyaluronan In Vitro," *Journal of the American Academy of Dermatology* 54, no. 3 (2006): 1124.

6. S. K. Katiyar, C. A. Elmets, R. Agarwal, J. Mukhtar, "Protection Against UVB Radiation—Induced Local and Systemic Suppression of Contact Hypersensitivity and Edema Responses in C3H/HeN Mice by Green Tea Polyphenols," *Photochemistry and Photobiology* 62, no. 5 (November 1995): 855–861.

7. Jaime L. Barger et al., "A Low Dose of Dietary Resveratrol Partially Mimics Caloric Restriction and Retards Aging Parameters in Mice" *PloS ONE* 3, no. 6 (June 2008): e2264.

8. Farrukh Afaq et al., "Prevention of Short-Term Ultraviolet B Radiation-mediated Damages by Resveratrol in SKH-1 Hairless Mice," *Toxicology and Applied Pharmacology* 186, no. 1 (January 2003): 28–37.

9. M. Seve, F. Chimienti, S. Devergnas, et al., "Resveratrol Enhances UVA-induced DNA Damage in HaCaT Human Keratinocytes," *Medicinal Chemistry* (Shariqah, United Arab Emirates), 2005 November:1(6): 629–633.

10. D. H. McDaniel et al., "Idebenone: A New Antioxidant—Part 1. Relative Assessment of Oxidative Stress Protection Capacity Compared to Commonly Known Antioxidants," *Journal of Cosmetic Dermatology* 4, no. 1 (January 2005): 10–17.

11. Joshua A. Tournas et al., "Ubiquinone, Idebenone, and Kinetin Provide Ineffective Photoprotection to Skin Compared to a Topical Antioxidant Combination of Vitamins C and E with Ferulic Acid," *Journal of Investigative Dermatology* 126, no. 5 (May 2006): 1185–1187.

12. D. McDaniel, B. Neudecker, J. DiNardo, et al., "Clinical Efficacy Assessment in Photodamaged Skin of 0.5% and 1.0% Idebenone," *Journal of Cosmetic Dermatology* 4, no. 3 (September 2005): 167–173.

13. G. Morissette, L. Germain, F. Marceau, "The Antiwrinkle Effect of Topical Concentrated 2-Dimethylaminoethanol Involves Vacuolar Cytopathology," *British Journal of Dermatology* 156, no. 3 (March 2007): 433–439.

14. A. Gragnani et al., "Dimethylaminoethanol Affects the Viability of Human Cultured Fibroblasts," *Aesthetic Plastic Surgery* 31, no. 6 November–December 2007): 711–718.

15. B. D. Gehm et al., "Resveratrol, a Polyphenolic Compound Found in Grapes and Wine, is an Agonist for the Estrogen Receptor," *Proceedings of the National Academy of Sciences of the United States of America* 94, no. 25 (December 1997): 14138–14143.

16. Eleanor G. Rogan, "Cancer Preventative Properties Identified in Resveratrol, Found in Red Wine, Red Grapes," *Science Daily* (July 2008).

CHAPTER 10 THE BIG BREAKTHROUGHS: COSMETIC PROCEDURES THAT DELIVER

1. F. Antonucci, C. Rossi, et al., "Long-Distance Retrograde Effects of Butulinum Neurotoxin A," *The Journal of Neuroscience* 28, no. 14 (April 2008): 3689–3696.
2. E. S. Marmur, R. Phelps, D. J. Goldberg, "Clinical, Histologic and Electron Microscopic Findings after Injection of a Calcium Hydroxylapatite Filler," *Journal of Cosmetic and Laser Therapy* 6, no. 4 (December 2004): 223–226.
3. C. M. Boyd, E. S. Marmur, S. C. Taylor, P. E. Grimes, and J. P. Porter, "Calcium Hydroxylapatite for Treatment of Nasolabial Folds in Persons of Color: Interim Safety Results at Three Months Post Injection," Accepted for publication in *Dermatologic Surgery*.

Index